AMERICAN
HEALTHCARE
REFORM

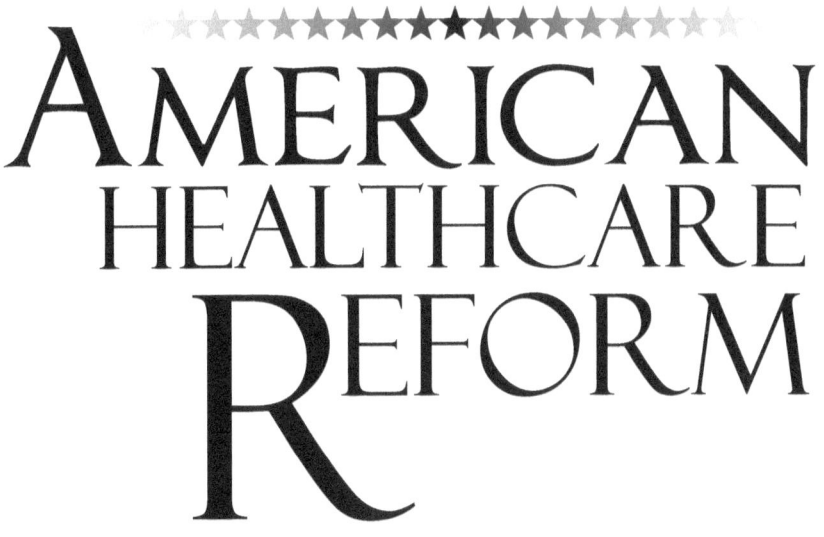

AMERICAN HEALTHCARE REFORM

Fixing The Real Problems

Earl W. Ferguson, MD, PhD

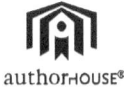

authorHOUSE®

AuthorHouse™ LLC
1663 Liberty Drive
Bloomington, IN 47403
www.authorhouse.com
Phone: 1-800-839-8640

Published by AuthorHouse 12/26/2013

ISBN: 978-1-4918-4315-4 (sc)
ISBN: 978-1-4918-4314-7 (hc)
ISBN: 978-1-4918-4313-0 (e)

Library of Congress Control Number: 2013923511

REVIEWS:

Dr. Ferguson has made a tremendous contribution to the current and future dialog concerning healthcare reform. From his broad experience across the spectrum of clinical care, research, government service and planning, he not only articulates well the problems and challenges our nation faces but offers sensible, data-based approaches to meaningful improvements and solutions. His historical perspective lends understanding to how we arrived at where we are and his knowledge of information technology, system processes and especially the psyche of the American people provide needed insights to both those deeply involved in various aspects of the healthcare system as well as to more casual, but interested, observers. This is a must read for anyone really interested in dealing with our current situation.

Cecil O. Samuelson, MD
President, Brigham Young University, Provo, Utah
Former Positions:
Professor of Internal Medicine; Dean, School of Medicine; Vice President, Health Sciences at the University of Utah
Senior Vice President, Intermountain Healthcare; President, Intermountain Healthcare Hospitals
Salt Lake City, Utah

American Healthcare Reform is a must read for all Americans interested in the future of United States healthcare. Dr. Earl Ferguson has written a logical, step-by-step analysis of the problems we have faced with the provision of healthcare in our nation as well as providing insightful solutions to correct multiple problems. Healthcare reform panic has gripped America and this book provides a map for ensuring quality of care at an effective cost in the future. What makes this book even more valuable is that it is written by a "real" medical doctor that has provided decades of care to his patients and also has been at the forefront of our rural health policy. His real stories and interview with other physicians and healthcare workers makes this an interesting, pertinent narrative. I highly recommend this book.

James Suver, MHA, Fellow American College of Healthcare Executives
CEO, Ridgecrest Regional Hospital
Adjunct Faculty, Department of Health and Community Services
California State University Chico

DEDICATION

To Sun Hye Paik, my best friend and wife
May we continue to work productively, enjoy life and
laugh every day in this great country of ours.

To my wonderful children and grandchildren
With the hope that our country will continue to give them the
same opportunities and challenges that it has given us.

CONTENTS

"Nothing in the world is more dangerous than sincere ignorance and conscientious stupidity"
—Martin Luther King, Jr.

PREFACE

This book was difficult to write for numerous reasons. First, the American healthcare system is highly complex, therefore, very difficult to understand. Second, the Affordable Care Act (ACA) of 2010 and its implementation are rapidly changing our healthcare system by adding more bureaucracies and regulatory requirements to a system that is already incomprehensible for most Americans. As additional bureaucracies are added, our healthcare system is continuing to become more complex, expensive and unaffordable. The senior Democratic Senator Max Baucus from Montana, Chair of the Senate Finance Committee, who was one of the major authors of the ACA, characterized the ACA as headed for a "train wreck." It is almost impossible to analyze a "train wreck" when we are in the middle of it. Third, public opinion on our healthcare system and how to reform it is highly polarized. That polarization is often driven by distorted or false information from highly partisan news and social media with opinions that are purposely one-sided. Fourth, political leaders and special interest groups and their leaders are exploiting these issues for political gain. We are not moving forward with compromises to find paths for meaningful and rational healthcare reform based on the data and capabilities that are available and ready for implementation.

This book will focus both on what is right and what is wrong with our uniquely American healthcare system. In truth, there is much that is right about our system, more than is wrong with it. The McKinsey Global Institute Report (*Accounting for the cost of US health care: A new look at why Americans spend more*, December 2008) defined the major issues of American healthcare costs. Many key issues are not what we usually hear from our political leadership and special interest groups. Before implementation of the ACA, Americans were healthier than the average of citizens in the 13 other developed Organization for Economic Cooperation and Development (OECD) peer countries. However, whether we get more value from the dollars we spend on healthcare is another issue. Of the $1.7 trillion we spent on healthcare in 2007, $477 billion was above expectations when compared with peer OECD countries. An estimated 21% of that excess spending was on health administration and our highly complex healthcare insurance system. Payments to hospitals and physicians accounted for most of the remaining excess spending and by far the largest portion was for outpatient services, including same-day hospital stays for surgeries and other procedures. The bulk of those payments went to hospitals and device manufacturers, not physicians.

We lead the world in medical innovations (development of drugs, medical devices, new procedures, etc.). We still believe and can demonstrate that the profit motive can drive both high quality and efficiency (cost-effectiveness) of healthcare. However, healthcare must be based on evidence-based, data-driven medicine. That requires transparency of data to evaluate performance and reduce unjustifiable variations in quality and costs. Timely information is essential for patients to make good decisions about their healthcare and for providers to continually improve our healthcare system. We should refocus on value and cost-effectiveness of care, not volume. We can do that by doing what we, as Americans do best—enabling and encouraging risk takers willing to invest their personal energy and money to develop innovative new products, services and systems of healthcare to move our country forward.

The profit motive is particularly important for driving innovations in healthcare. It can and should be harnessed correctly as a force for delivery of high quality, cost-effective healthcare services, as well as for keeping our population healthy by promoting wellness, health promotion and preventive medicine services with incentives for all our citizens. Changing our uniquely American healthcare system to a totally socialized system, rather than the public-private partnership that we already have, is not the answer.

Socialized medicine has many definitions that we should understand in considering the system we currently have and comparing it to the systems in other countries. Socialized medicine can be a government-operated healthcare system that employs healthcare providers. The British National Health Service (NHS) is an example, as are the US military healthcare and Veterans Administration healthcare systems. A broader definition of socialized medicine includes government financing of healthcare services without direct provision of those services. The Canadian healthcare system and those of most Western European countries (our peer OECD countries) deliver care through partial or total funding of public or public-private partnership systems. We do the same with Medicare, Medicaid and the US military TRICARE insurance.

One of the best examples of a rational, well-designed and relatively efficient national healthcare system is that of France. France has universal coverage for all citizens and reimburses 70% of most medical expenses (Edmonds, M "10 Health Care Systems Around the World" 2013 people. howstuffworks.com/10-health-care-systems.htm). Patients can see anyone they choose and 42% of the time they can get a same-day appointment (Cohn, J "Healthy Examples" *Boston Globe* July 5, 2009, www.boston. com). In 2000, the World Health Organization (WHO) ranked France first in its survey of healthcare systems. Patients pay their share up front for the care so they are aware of the costs, encouraging them to use the system wisely. France also focuses on health promotion and preventive medicine with complete, free checkups every five years and incentives for prenatal care for low-income patients, as well as care for children. Life expectancies are greater than 80 years and costs for healthcare are half those in the US (*Health at a Glance 2011: OECD Indicators*, www.oecd. org/els/health-systems49105858.pdf). However, even France is a mixture of public and private systems. The vast majority of the French people purchase private insurance to cover their share of the costs.

The bottom line in these examples is that we already operate a public-private healthcare system in the US. We do not have "universal healthcare" or "public healthcare" for all our citizens, but we have covered the vast majority of our citizens, including low income and underserved populations, before the ACA. Our biggest problems have been those people who chose not to get healthcare insurance. The important question is how can we provide truly affordable healthcare more effectively and efficiently for most or all of our citizens without markedly increasing the costs and still allow health insurance choices for most Americans? When we have answered that important question, we can begin making rational changes to reform our healthcare system in meaningful ways.

Meaningful healthcare reform requires understanding of our complex healthcare system. This book was written to help clarify the difficult and poorly understood issues and problems of American healthcare. Its purpose is to help us move forward on the many difficult decisions that should be made to improve our healthcare system. Our unique combination of public-private funding and free-market capitalism has been a major source of medical care advancements over the last half-century. The entrepreneurial spirit of risk takers who have invested billions of dollars to push forward innovative ideas and products has been key to its success. We should not lose that driving force for medical advancements and our economy.

Our American healthcare system needs reform. We should fix it rationally with a scalpel, not destroy it with a meat cleaver. To optimize and appropriately guide that reform, we should first understand and concentrate on the real problems. Primarily we should fix our healthcare system by decreasing its administrative complexity and inefficiencies. The Accountable Care Act should be modified significantly to make it more acceptable as part of our national effort for more meaningful reform. Rational solutions through political compromises are not easy to find in our highly polarized political environment. It will be a long uphill climb, but it is a challenge that we must meet for our uniquely American healthcare system to survive.

"I have only one yardstick by which I test every major problem—and that yardstick is: Is it good for America?"
—Dwight D. Eisenhower

AUTHOR'S PERSPECTIVE

I wrote this book from the perspective of a career public servant. I'm a retired Air Force medical officer and a cardiologist in solo practice in an isolated, rural area. I have learned the difficulties of providing healthcare in both well-supported and austere environments. I've also had the opportunity to observe and study many different aspects of our healthcare system and our sociocultural diversities, as well as the healthcare systems and cultures of many other countries. Growing up in the military and then serving as a medical officer, I have received my healthcare from our military healthcare system most of my life. I have also worked with Veterans Administration Hospitals. I like to think of our US military healthcare system as one of the largest and most experienced health maintenance organizations (HMOs) in the world, providing excellent care.

My experience as a medical officer was diverse. The first half of my military career was in academic medicine at the Uniformed Services University of the Health Sciences in Bethesda, Maryland. The last half of my Federal service career was in senior executive management in military medical centers, hospitals, and larger health systems, and then with NASA as the Director of Aerospace Medicine and Occupational Health.

I left Federal service in 1996 to join a small rural primary care practice in Ridgecrest, California, to develop telemedicine, computer and other advanced health information technology for healthcare in remote underserved areas. In that practice I learned the realities of our non-Federal American healthcare system, including the business of medicine and fee-for-service practice. My experience in private practice and my work on boards and in leadership positions of many not-for-profit organizations that focused on rural health and the application of innovative technologies taught me much about the tremendous complexities and the many problems of our current system.

Looking at our healthcare development and problems, I see many analogies to how airplanes are designed, built and tested. "Pushing the envelope" is a test pilot term for pushing an aircraft's performance beyond the known performance limits for safe flight. Pushing the envelope is necessary to learn how to adjust and increase aircraft performance limits with new innovations. Test pilots do that very methodically with gradually increasing excursions outside the envelope ("outside the box"). That is where we are now going with healthcare reform—pushing the envelope—but we are not doing it in the same incremental and relatively "safe" manner that test pilots employ. Test pilots would not take a newly designed airplane through the sound barrier on its first flight, even with extensive knowledge of every system and the designed performance limits. Our healthcare system is much more complex than a newly designed airplane. We should not push critically needed healthcare reform too far and too fast outside the envelope where the risks of catastrophic failure are very high.

Our decisions should be based on sound, data-supported information that appears to be correct, even if those decisions go against prevailing opinion and are politically sensitive. This often requires addressing controversial issues. Thinking outside the box and pushing the envelope is an exciting and interesting way to stimulate change and to travel through life. It is not without hazards and it requires being simultaneously comfortable and uncomfortable with risks—knowing the balance at the edge of the envelope. It also requires the ability to adapt to data that proves to be contrary to initial expectations, as well as to adjust opinions to reach necessary consensus and compromises.

As a scientist, I have spent a significant portion of my research career disproving many of my pet hypotheses. That is what research is all about. If everything worked out as it "should" based on what we know already and all our logical hypotheses were correct, we would not need to do research. However, many times, if not most of the time, logical hypotheses prove to be wrong. We should have faith in reason and inquiry, embrace doubt and be skeptical of "certainty". Evaluating and investigating issues with an open mind takes us down paths that can lead us to important discoveries that we do not expect.

Chance also provides unexpected opportunities that can also lead us to interesting career paths (or educational diversions) on "the roads less travelled." Flying a glider (sailplane) in Maryland in the early 1980s led to conversations with Les Gawlik, JD, Solicitor for the Mayor and City Council of Baltimore. Les was involved in a lawsuit regarding the Age Discrimination in Employment Act of 1967 (ADEA) and firefighters employed by the city. The ADEA prohibits employers from discrimination based on age for employees ages 40 to 70 by discharging them or requiring them to retire involuntarily, except where age is a "bona fide occupational qualification (BFOQ) reasonably necessary to the normal operation of a particular business." Les asked for my opinion when he learned that I was a cardiologist and exercise physiologist and was doing research on human performance at the Uniformed Services University of the Health Sciences, Bethesda, Maryland. In our initial discussions, I told him that the law appeared to be clear that such discrimination was not consistent with the ADEA and that I could test anyone's capability to perform their job by exercise testing and other performance standards.

Les was persistent and over several weeks educated me more about what the BFOQ provision meant. Eventually he brought me interesting statistics related to deaths in firefighters. In 1978, of 162 firefighter deaths reported to the National Fire Protection Association, 72 (44.4%) were from heart attacks. More than half of those deaths were during firefighting activities and many were thought to be stress-related. There were similar statistics from 1979. Based on that information, I agreed to look further into the problem and spent time with the firefighters in Baltimore to learn more about their activities and stresses. That experience and further literature review convinced me that a BFOQ of age 55 could be justified. Published data demonstrated that the risk of heart attacks in firefighters was significantly higher than in the general population and that the risk of heart attacks increased markedly after age 55. If a firefighter had a heart attack while fighting a fire it could put the public safety at risk, as well as put that firefighter's partner at risk because firefighters work in pairs if they are inside of a burning building.

I agreed to help Les with his case, as an expert witness in the Federal District Court in Baltimore. The Court held that the city had failed to make its case for the BFOQ defense. I published my opinion on the risks of undetected heart disease in firefighters and the inability to detect that disease with routine exercise stress testing (Ferguson, E "Detection of coronary artery disease in fire fighters without symptoms: Routine exercise testing is inadequate" *Firechief* (1981) 47:14-17). I subsequently moved out of Maryland and lost touch with Les.

However, two military assignments later, when I was Chief of Staff, USAF Medical Center Scott, in Illinois, I received a call from Colonel Clinton Pagano, Superintendent, Department of Law and Public Safety, State of New Jersey. He informed me that he had been trying to find me because of my *Firechief* article that was included in the Supreme Court records after the decision on the Baltimore case (EEOC v. Baltimore, 472 U.S. 353, 105 S.Ct. 2717, 86 L.Ed.2d 286, 1985). Col Pagano wanted my help on establishing a physical fitness program and physical fitness standards for the New Jersey State Police. He felt that the program was essential for the health of his troopers and also necessary to justify retirement of those officers at age 55 that he thought would be challenged by the Equal Employment Opportunity Commission (EEOC). I helped Col Pagano and his staff set up those programs. The EEOC filed suit against the State of New Jersey, New Jersey State Police and went to trial. I testified as an expert witness and the decision was for support of age 55 as a BFOQ, relying heavily on the facts I presented (EEOC v. State of N.J., 631 F.Supp. 1506 (1986)). These and other experiences got me even more interested in the prevention and management of risks of early coronary artery disease, public policy, the law and other related issues. When I was Commander, USAF Little Rock Hospital, Arkansas, I attended night school at the University of Arkansas School of Law at Little Rock, to learn more about the law, but was soon moved on to another assignment. Even that brief experience was invaluable in increasing my understanding of legal ethics, how lawyers think, and how they approach cases.

One final point is, facts and the data available to make healthcare decisions evolve over time. We must, therefore, adjust our thinking about how to manage healthcare and other issues. As an example, coronary artery disease risks have evolved significantly over the last few decades. As a country we have been focusing more on healthy lifestyles and decreasing risks from hypertension, smoking, elevated cholesterol, sedentary lifestyle, etc. We have markedly decreased the number of deaths from acute coronary artery events, although they are still the biggest healthcare issue in our country. In addition, for the first time we are developing technologies that may allow us to detect and treat early coronary disease to prevent problems decades before the onset of significant disease. Risks of sudden death from asymptomatic (without symptoms) coronary artery disease in apparently healthy individuals may be detected earlier with new biomarkers that are currently being studied and developed. Instead of classic biomarkers of late disease, such as calcium scores (an index of calcification in the coronary arteries), the future will be in biomarkers to diagnose very early atherosclerotic cardiovascular disease (ASCVD). Emerging systems biology approaches that include gene and protein responses to any disease will enable personalized medical interventions and treatments designed specifically for each patient. Those biomarkers and cardiac computer tomography angiography (CCTA) in selected individuals, such as firefighters and pilots, may allow them to work at higher ages without major risks of sudden cardiac death that could jeopardize public safety. All these healthcare issues must be managed based on the realities of current data, the medical technologies available and our ability to make good, clear decisions. This is the same rational, evidence-based way we should approach healthcare reform and healthcare policy.

"The danger posed by the growing power of the administrative state cannot be dismissed."
—Chief Justice John Roberts

INTRODUCTION

What is wrong with American healthcare?

There are several basic problems that are the major sources of dissatisfaction with our American healthcare system.

First, Federal and state governments, big healthcare businesses and special interest groups now drive and manipulate the supply and demand for healthcare services. The responsiveness of our healthcare system to patients, to families, to healthcare providers, and to free market forces has been markedly distorted by special interests and their influences on our politicians and Federal and state bureaucracies.

Second, healthcare delivery has evolved from a service to an enormous business consuming approximately 18% of our gross domestic product (GDP) and continuing to grow rapidly. The current healthcare environment has pressured physicians and other healthcare providers to move more toward the assembly line mentality of business. Focusing more on business plans and/or joining hospital networks or other larger practice networks are strategies that many healthcare provider practices have followed or considered for survival. The complexity of regulatory compliance and risk of failures to meet every letter of laws, rules and regulations in reimbursement procedures is overwhelming providers. It is diverting a large amount of their time away from actually providing healthcare to patients. We should get providers back to concentrating on the service of providing high quality healthcare that is the major generator of professional satisfaction. We should relieve them from excessive, bureaucratic administrative and business burdens.

Third, patients and healthcare providers are being forced to live with rules made by people who are far removed from providing care. Government overregulation and insurance company administrative requirements are overwhelming patients and healthcare providers, increasing the complexity of healthcare delivery and generating excessive administrative costs.

Why is American healthcare so expensive?

In addition to the basic overarching problems listed above, there are other specific reasons for high healthcare costs, including:

- *Excessive utilization of expensive new drugs and innovative technologies, including many that add little or no incremental value (or even prove to be harmful) and are not cost-effective,*
- *Manipulation of the supply of healthcare providers,* i.e., training programs, immigration, scope of licensing issues, etc.,
- *Manipulation of the demand for services* by mass marketing of expensive brand name drugs, technologies and services directly to patients and consumers, as well as providers,
- *Lack of comprehensive disease prevention programs* focused on health and wellness that can decrease the risk of expensive, debilitating diseases,
- *Lack of adequate chronic disease management services, including comprehensive mental health services,* focused on total care of patients with the highest costs for frequent hospitalizations, re-hospitalizations and emergency department visits, and costly procedures,
- *Excessive use of laboratory testing and procedures,* often driven by fear of malpractice litigation, a much bigger problem in the many states that have not instituted adequate malpractice tort reform,
- *High costs of end-of-life care* from overutilization of intensive care, ventilators, imaging, multiple hospitalizations, and other heroic measures for many patients with little or no chance of recovery and no expectancy of prolonged meaningful life,
- *Minimal or no significant healthcare cost-sharing for many patients,* providing no incentive for cost-savings,
- *Failure of patients and families to take responsibility for their own health* and failure of governmental and non-governmental

organizations to adequately foster that responsibility in our society.

- *Disproportionately high reimbursement for procedures, compared to preventive and chronic care.*

How is the Affordable Care Act of 2010 affecting changes in our current healthcare system?

The origins of the Affordable Care Act (ACA) of 2010 were skeletal guidelines for healthcare reform by staffers of senior Democratic Senator Max Baucus from Montana, Chair of the Senate Finance Committee, and senior Republican Senator Chuck Grassley from Iowa, Member of the Senate Finance Committee and Ranking Republican Member of the Senate Judiciary Committee, three years before the ACA. Those guidelines did not focus on specific strategies, because specifics would have made it difficult, if not impossible, to craft healthcare reform legislation. The basic idea was to let "us" develop its implementation. Therefore, the final details of the ACA were crafted without adequate oversight and review.

Despite the way this legislation was forced through Congress, the ACA and the Health Information Technology for Economic and Clinical Health (HITECH) Act have pushed for many positive changes that many can agree on:

- More universal healthcare insurance coverage,
- Insurance for pre-existing conditions,
- No lifetime maximum for healthcare costs,
- Implementation of electronic health records (EHRs) and advanced health information technology (HIT) systems, although they are still far from meeting adequate usability and interoperability standards,
- New systems of care (Patient Centered Medical Homes, Accountable Care Organizations, etc.) to improve coordination of our personal healthcare and programs for disease prevention, with documentation of quality and cost-effectiveness of care.

However, the promise of more transparency regarding costs and options for services and procedures to allow patients to make

3

more informed decisions is becoming less and less apparent with the implementation of the ACA. Many are concerned with the marked increases in costs of healthcare with the implementation of the ACA and with the cancellation of millions of healthcare insurance policies that policyholders were satisfied with and were told they could keep. The increases in insurance costs are driven by the mandates for more uniform and comprehensive healthcare insurance policies and for "essential" benefits that many do not want or need. Those mandates are increasing everyone's health insurance costs. Other irritants that are grossly unfair are the special exemptions that the ACA gave to members of Congress and Federal government workers with highly subsidized "Cadillac" plans and the temporary administrative exemptions that are being given to big businesses and other special interest groups, but not the general public.

Other major issues include the failures of the information technology systems required to coordinate the implementation of the ACA. The Federal health information exchange system for enrolling patients in the healthcare insurance system (Healthcare.gov website) was a greater than $500M disaster. Even more critically, the information technology systems necessary for the "meaningful use" of data in electronic health records (EHRs) and the healthcare information exchange (HIE) systems needed to move that data among different systems to effectively coordinate care are far from ready for wide implementation.

Monitoring and feedback on the quality and efficiency of our healthcare system will require implementation of health information technology (HIT) systems that are still not adequately developed, usable and interoperable. Nevertheless, the Health Information Technology for Economic and Clinical Health (HITECH) Act that was part of the American Recovery and Reinvestment Act (ARRA) of 2009 and ACA should be acknowledged for elevating HIT implementation and healthcare reform to prominent positions on America's agenda. In particular, the HITECH Act pushed implementation of EHRs for more meaningful use of health information technologies and more open exchange of healthcare information. This is highly positive. However, there was also a negative side to how this was implemented. Providers were forced to begin making decisions on selection of EHR systems before the Office of the National Coordinator (ONC) for Health Information Technology of the Department of Health and Human Services (DHHS) certified them. In fact, the hundreds of EHRs certified and currently on the market were only certified for minimal functionality (Audit logs, e-Prescribing, PQRS reports, etc.). In addition, the most implemented EHR products certified by ONC have failed to meet usability and interoperability expectations. As will be discussed in this book, pushing for automation of healthcare processes before those processes are fully examined, understood, simplified and standardized is problematic. We can't fix the broken administrative and bureaucratic processes that existed even before the ACA by simply automating them with advanced HIT systems, especially if we are adding EHR systems that lack adequate usability and interoperability.

"Even small health care institutions are complex, barely manageable places. Large health care organizations may be the most complex organizations in human history."—Peter Drucker

Healthcare Costs: History and Perspective

How did so many problems develop with our healthcare system?

Major factors in the transformation of American healthcare from a profession to a business, and the resultant explosion of costs include: The Social Security Act of 1965, physician and attorney advertising, increased costs of medical education, increased time in post-graduate specialty training, changes in the professional expectations of newly trained physicians, implementation of innovative healthcare technologies, increased administrative and reporting requirements, excessive regulatory burdens, advertising of pharmaceuticals and products directly to patients, legal risks (malpractice and class action suits and regulatory compliance risks), end-of-life care, and failure of individuals and families to take responsibility for their own health.

Healthcare reform requires dealing with many complex issues. The issues are highly political, emotional, and strongly supported by special interest groups, making them difficult to resolve and improve productively. They should be addressed with detailed studies to reach compromises based on clearly defined, objective data. Focusing on basic general principles, socioeconomic goals, and values that we can agree or compromise on and support are the only way to move this discussion forward.

Governmental healthcare legislation, rules, regulations and policies, as well as third party payer rules and policies, are always slow to change.

Reforming healthcare bureaucracies—lowering barriers and simplifying processes—will be difficult.

Social Security Act of 1965: Implementation of Medicare and Medicaid under the Social Security Act of 1965 provided healthcare insurance to a large number of patients and paid physicians for services that were previously provided through private insurance, personal pay or charity care. It markedly improved physician incomes and was *the major step in government funding that began the transition of healthcare from a profession to a very expensive, largely government-funded business.* However, it has proven to be the most successful public-private healthcare insurance program in American history.

Attorney and physician advertising: Prohibition of advertising was a basic tenet of both the legal and medical profession. The first American Medical Association Code of Ethics in 1847 prohibited physicians from advertising. In 1975 the Federal Trade Commission (FTC) accused the legal and medical professions of restraint of trade. *In 1976 the US Supreme Court decision that allowed lawyers to advertise started the erosion of these basic professional tenets.*

Changes in medical education: The expenses of medical school, increases in the length of post-graduate medical education and in medical practice specialization, along with cultural changes, have markedly altered the professional expectations of newly trained physicians. Medical training in the US includes a four-year college degree, four years of medical school, and generally three to five or more years of specialty training, depending on specialty and sub-specialty. Even general practice (primary care practices of family practice, general internal medicine and pediatrics) now requires specialty training. Most other developed countries provide free medical education, but in the US it is expensive and must be paid for by individuals and their families or by scholarships and loans. Physicians finish their basic medical school training with large debts. Median costs for medical school graduates in 2011 were $264,000 for private schools and $187,400 for public schools; median debts were $180,000 for private schools and $155,000 for public schools (Youngclaus, J, *Analysis in Brief* 12(2) July 2012, Association of American Medical Colleges). New physicians entering practice must focus on repaying those debts, in addition to the costs of opening a practice. Many choose to join large practices in urban areas, rather than starting their own practices, particularly in rural areas. They must focus on the business of medical practice and their expectations are six figure incomes to pay for their investments of the more than 10-years in training.

Until the 1970s and 1980s, post-graduate medical training (residencies for "residents"—called residents because medical trainees previously lived in the hospital or on the hospital grounds) was very intense and traditionally required long hours in the hospital taking care of patients. I was a product of that training and feel that it served me well. When I finished my general internal medicine training in 1973, I was confident that I could deal with difficult medical issues—including knowing how to rapidly think through complex problems and where to go for help when I needed it.

Starting in the 1970s, residency on-call hours were decreased because of concerns that sleep deprivation increased medical errors. This began a major change in American post-graduate medical training. In July 2003 the Accreditation Council for Graduate Medical Education (ACGME) limited the number of work-hours for residents to 80 hours a week (averaged over four weeks), no more than every third night on-call, and 10 hours off between shifts. In July 2011 the ACGME further limited first-year residents to 16-hour shifts and the number of new patients they could manage ("work-up" with history, physical, assessment of problems and plan for management) during those shifts. A Mayo Clinic study concluded that the limitation made residents feel less prepared for management of their patients, especially the increased transfer of care from one provider to another, after the change was imposed (Prep, V. "A Review of Studies on Medical Residency Work Hour Changes" *U.S. News & World Report* September 12, 2013). Other studies have found the data on this change inconclusive. To compensate for fewer work hours, the length of residency training (and consequently its expense) has increased. *However, intensity of experience may be more important for learning than generally acknowledged and increased time in residency may not be adequate to provide equivalent training.*

The changes in training, professional expectations, lifestyle and family expectations have been particularly devastating for rural healthcare. Over the last few years, more and more graduates (about a quarter) are selecting the primary care specialties of internal medicine, family practice, and pediatrics (USA Today, March 15, 2013). This is an important trend because we need more primary care specialists for better healthcare coordination requiring primary care specialists. However, newly trained primary care physicians often prefer to live in large cities and join urban group practices. This can decrease their business uncertainties and their financial and administrative burdens. In addition, many young internal medicine and family physicians who move to practices in rural areas often choose to see patients in clinic for a fixed number of hours (usually less than six hours of patient care) a day and no more than five days a week with no call (nighttime coverage of practice), or to be hospitalists and not see patients in clinic. This is a different practice pattern than older rural practitioners who provide full-care services for their patients (both clinic and hospital care).

Factors in these decisions may include less rigorous post-graduate medical education, more interest in quality-of-life issues and the move from fee-for-service practices to salaried or hourly rate practices. *Private, fee-for-service practices are generally more efficient than community clinics with salaried practitioners because of the profit motive for productivity.* There is nothing as effective as appropriate financial incentives for driving productivity and high quality, cost-effective healthcare.

Development of innovative healthcare technologies: American healthcare is exceptional and is the envy of the world. Many citizens of other countries come to the US for healthcare because we have been innovative in the development and application of new technologies and drugs. Innovation is the highly positive side of our healthcare system that has historically set us apart from other healthcare systems. Research and development of drugs, medical devices, and related healthcare innovations should be encouraged and supported by government grants and private investments.

However, innovation has its negatives. *Overutilization of expensive technologies, such as imaging technologies and procedures, has become the standard of care.* It is amazing how many expensive studies a large number of patients have had—multiple CTs, nuclear studies, MRIs, ultrasound studies, etc., not just routine X-rays. *Overutilization of technologies is a major factor in high healthcare costs, driven by defensive medicine to avoid the risk of malpractice litigation, by reimbursement for procedures, and by patient demands and expectations.*

Overuse of technologies is a major area of review. Strong recommendations have been made and should continue to be made regarding the appropriateness and evidence-based indications for these studies, especially those driven by fee-for-service motives. Other factors include *direct advertising of new drugs and procedures to providers and the public.* They are often not cost-effective, adding little incremental benefit when compared with standard and more proven alternatives. In many cases, these new drugs and procedures actually prove to be more harmful alternatives than previous practices. A review of all 363 original articles comparing innovations with standard practices published in the *New England Journal of Medicine* from 2001-2010 found that 40.2% of the innovations were no better than standard practices (but are often much more expensive), 38.0% of innovations were confirmed as superior, and comparisons were inconclusive in 21.8% of the studies (*Mayo Clin Proc.* 2013: 88(8): 790-798). Only 38% of innovations were improvements in care compared with more standard, generally much less expensive alternatives.

There is a critical need for continued comparison of new practices with standard ones to support evidence-based decisions. Innovations in evidence-based decision-making, such as the "cognitive computing" capabilities of IBM's Watson computer and other data analysis "learning" programs, have the potential to markedly improve complex healthcare data management. This can move us toward better overall healthcare system management, as well as more patient-specific evidence-based medical decisions and personalized medicine (Hempel, J, "IBM's Massive Bet on Watson" *Fortune* (October 7, 2013) 168(6): 80).

We should also focus on clinical practice innovation, including more comprehensive coordinated care for patients with chronic diseases using teams of primary care providers, mid-level providers (nurse practitioners and physician assistants), nurses, social workers, care coordinators and other specialists. The opportunities for patient-centered clinical practice innovations, such as Accountable Care Organizations (ACOs) and Coordinated Care Organizations (CCOs) have the potential to make a major difference in quality and cost-effectiveness of healthcare delivery and promotion of the general health of communities. Innovations to be considered for better care coordination include emergency departments (EDs) specifically for geriatric patients, better coordination of patient load and flow for scheduled surgeries (Litvak, E, and H V Fineberg

"Smoothing the Way to High Quality, Safety, and Economy" *N Engl J Med* (October 24, 2013) 369;17: 1581-1583), and early training of undergraduates interested in healthcare careers as volunteer Health Coaches to assist patients with compliance on medications and other health issues in their homes (Barry Bittman, MD, Senior Fellow, Estes Park Institute, presentations Monterey, CA October 21-23, 2013).

Administrative, reporting and other requirements: *Rising clinical provider overhead costs, largely driven by continued increases in Federal, state, and insurance company record-keeping, administrative, reporting and other requirements, are devastating single provider and small group practices. Increases in costs to meet mandated administrative and regulatory requirements are already excessive.* Efficient clinical practices employ an average of 3.5 full-time equivalents (FTEs) for every provider to manage their offices. Nationwide median reimbursement for primary care providers in 2009 was $504,169 total medical revenue with total operating costs of $294,360 (58% of revenue) (Medical Group Management Association Cost Survey for Primary Care Practices 2010 Report Based on 2009 Data). This course for our healthcare system is unsustainable, but new regulatory, record keeping and administrative requirements continue to be added. These requirements must be simplified to decrease the burden on healthcare providers.

The high administrative costs are critical in the light of potential additional cuts of physician reimbursement. With high administrative and overhead costs of >50%, further cuts in Medicare and Medicaid reimbursements would actually cut provider income (take home pay) by 20 to 40% or more. In addition, reimbursement for specialty care was already reduced administratively in 2012 by the Medicare/Medicaid (CMS) decision to delete billing codes for specialty consults. Only allowing billing for routine visits decreased reimbursement for specialty consults by as much as 22%. These issues are driving many specialty providers and other providers to retire early or leave the clinical practice of medicine.

The push for EHR system adoption and meaningful use is also problematic. Many physicians and physician groups have examined the business case for proceeding with later stages of HIE meaningful use requirements. Since meeting those requirements will be expensive both in terms of hardware, software and administrative costs, a significant number are reluctant to proceed further. Without further incentives they feel that the penalties will be less expensive than implementing those systems or they will choose to retire or leave the practice of medicine.

My younger brother, a recently retired rural family practice physician, proponent of a single payer system and supporter of the ACA, commented on his frustrations with EHRs and HIE documentation requirements:

> ". . . the EHR helps automate a lot of it. It is mostly a pain and interferes with the flow of patient care and does little to improve it. I resent having to include a complex series of codes to every visit just so some administrative bean counter can find a way to justify not paying me. The claim that tracking these codes will improve care or improve research is untrue. This type of data mining will not provide scientifically valid research. If they want to do research, set up and pay for a study. Don't impose requirements on thousands of providers. Education of providers and patients has always been the best way to improve care."

He also had a perspective on "meaningful use" that is instructive—

> "Anyone who goes to the trouble of using an EHR and sticks with it will be making 'meaningful use' of it. I have been meaningfully using an EHR for ten years. I agree with a lot of the intent of the CMS definition of 'meaningful use', but think it should be very basic and easy to achieve. The providers who stick to their EHR will evolve with the progression of the whole system."

These issues do not just involve physicians. I talked with a vocational rehabilitation counselor from Oregon who experienced difficult problems with getting people to do the right thing and take care of themselves. Unfortunately, she said that she always has to focus on negatives with no time to focus on positives and prevention. She said that 80% of her time was spent verifying disabilities, documentation, data entry and policy and procedures. She could only spend 20% of her time face-to-face with clients. She was looking for other career options—"I too am out the door."

Other excessive regulatory burdens: Jumping through the regulatory hoops for hospital construction, clinic construction, and construction of healthcare support infrastructures, such as broadband to rural areas is excessively time-consuming, complicated and expensive. Major projects can be delayed or halted altogether by required environmental impact statements and other requirements that have pushed expenses far beyond what should be considered reasonable.

In California, for example, the Office for Statewide Health Planning and Development (OSHPD), must approve all aspects of hospital construction (California is not a certificate-of-need state). Ridgecrest Regional Hospital, where I practice and where I am a Board member, just completed a major hospital renovation. I watched the construction progress and noted some unusual activities. For example, a trench was dug through our Emergency Department driveway where pipes were laid, then the trench backfilled with concrete, sand and blacktop. When another trench was dug right next to the previous trench and more pipe was laid and similarly backfilled a week or so later, I asked our local contractor overseeing the construction why both piping jobs could not have been done in the same trench. The answer was that OSHPD would not approve starting the second piping job until the first one was complete, including sealing and blacktop.

In mid-2011, our hospital committed to purchasing a $2M CT imaging system to improve services and offer new programs, including rapid evaluation of coronary artery disease by coronary CT angiography in people with chest pain. Such a program could decrease by more than 85% the need to transfer patients with chest pain to larger hospitals, a two-hour ambulance ride away, for invasive diagnostic coronary angiography, and markedly improve the care of patients in our isolated region (see Poon, M, *et al. J Am Coll Cardiol* 2013;62:543-52). We identified a room in our Radiology Department to house the system. Renovations for that room were projected to cost less than $100,000 and qualified for an expedited OSHPD review. Rapid approval was expected. However, the extended negotiations with OSHPD took more than two years for approval to install the CT and we had to hire a construction firm to help us with the application process. One of the interesting OSHPD requirements was that a payphone be located near the room. Since cellphones are now used extensively, our local phone company no longer installs payphones. To get the project approved we had to put in a payphone and give the local phone company a monthly guarantee for its use and it is fairly certain that the phone will never be used. There were many other delaying issues raised by OSHPD that had little merit when weighed against our community needs. There appears to be no sense of urgency with regard for critical patient care and community priorities. To try to push this along faster, in July 2013 we talked to the architectural firm overseeing this process about the advisability of talking to OSHPD directly or going to one of our legislators. We got this response:

> "We understand and share your frustration, but we are not sure either approach will help the situation. We contacted the Rapid Review supervisor, (name deleted), and she agreed to do what she can to expedite the review. It's currently scheduled to be completed by 8-27-13, but she said some of the team is ahead of schedule and could be done sooner. We agreed to follow up next week on the status. *I'm more skeptical about the success of getting a legislator involved as it will complicate things, irritate them, and may result in further delays, if not on this item then others. It is not in our interests to create friction with them unnecessarily as it is an ongoing relationship.* (italics added)
> They are unable to schedule an Over-The-Counter (OTC) review due to the volume of submittals to address, but we may be able to communicate with the reviewers directly to clear their comments. We will check back with them next week on the status, if we don't hear from them sooner. We will keep you informed of the progress."

The bottom line on this project is that we spent over two years and $400,000 just to get approval to make renovations expected to cost less than $100,000. An architectural contractor who felt intimidated by OSHPD made numerous changes in plans required by multiple reviews at OSHPD that resulted in delays in a project that would markedly improve patient care and save millions of dollars in healthcare costs by avoiding transfers out of our area. Installation of our CT is now not expected until 2014, almost three years after we made the decision to install the CT. Is such bureaucratic inefficiency and obstruction the way to improve the quality and cost-effectiveness of our healthcare system and decrease healthcare costs? OSHPD's intent is noteworthy—we want safe hospitals. However, its inflexibility and impractical standards prevent or impede progress.

More recently, our hospital decreased the number of acute care beds to become a critical access hospital (CAH), limited to 25 acute care beds. It was our best option for financial survival in the current economic and healthcare climate. Our application was made through the California Health and Human Services (CHHS) Department of Public Health (DPH). A copy of that application was available online, but it could not be downloaded, printed, filled-out and submitted, because DPH required that it be submitted on a specially colored paper that had to be mailed to the hospital. Our Ridgecrest Regional Hospital administration had to wait two months for the application and finally had to get the California Hospital Association, Office of Rural Health Policy, and a California legislator involved before it was sent. The Kern County DPH Office in Bakersfield, a two-hour drive away, said that they were "too busy" to respond to our request. This is not the way to efficiently run a healthcare system to meet the needs of underserved rural communities.

Another issue is that by California law, hospitals cannot employ physicians. Large healthcare systems can create medical foundations and hire physicians through those foundations. However, this is not an option for many small rural hospitals and district hospitals. This markedly decreases their ability to attract physicians to rural areas where they are critically needed.

The last issue on excessive regulation and government bureaucracies is a more general problem. Broadband information technologies are desperately needed in remote areas to provide services for underserved populations, not just healthcare providers. I am one of the Directors of the California Broadband Collaborative (CBC) that has responsibility for oversight of the $81M federally funded Broadband Technologies Opportunities Program (BTOP) Digital 395 Project matched with $28M from the California Advanced Services Fund (totaling $111M including private funds). The Project laid approximately 600 miles of fiber optic cable, supporting gigabyte services, to hospitals and more than 300 other institutions and service providers. This will support 45,000 commercial and residential customers occupying 12% of the total land area of California. The route mainly follows Highway 395 from Barstow, CA, to Reno, NV, through the isolated, rural, high-desert area of California east of the Sierras. It will markedly improve our HIT capabilities and the general healthcare for residents of these regions, as well as stimulating economic development in these underserved areas.

I was amazed at the complexity of legal, environmental, regulatory and political barriers to complete this project. In the end, the biggest expense (approaching $30M) was dealing with legal, environmental, regulatory and permit issues satisfying requirements from more than 50 oversight agencies, with much of those expenses being paid back to or involving the Federal government.

Simplifying the bureaucratic processes that markedly delay implementation of urgently needed, cost-effective, innovative technologies with proven benefits is as important a priority for healthcare as funding. The administrative, regulatory, legal, and political burdens that must be surmounted to get anything done in this country, in California, and in many other states have become major barriers to progress in any project or major economic undertaking. Many individuals in government agencies try very hard to assist us with critical services and express their frustration with the difficulties they have in effectively accomplishing their jobs. The bureaucratic barriers have grown far beyond any reasonable expectation and have led to a stagnated system that is always slow and often totally unable or unwilling to respond. They make projects so expensive that they have become a major threat to economic progress in our country. Well meaning government workers are often so hampered by the bureaucracy of laws, rules and regulations that they are not permitted to make simple decisions based on common sense. There appears to be no political will or understanding of the need to make the hard decisions that are necessary to reduce these crippling administrative and bureaucratic burdens. We must, somehow, put some certainty and hope back into businesses and our economy by focusing on long-term stable solutions that decrease costs and simplify our excessively bureaucratic processes. These issues extend far beyond healthcare.

Direct advertising to patients: The US and New Zealand are the only countries that allow direct advertising of pharmaceuticals and other medical products to consumers (patients and their families). *Direct-to-consumer advertising (DTCA) of pharmaceuticals is banned in more than 30 other industrialized nations.* In recent years, mass media advertisement for pharmaceuticals to consumers in the US has markedly increased. Spending on direct-to-consumer advertising quadrupled from less than $1.0B in 1997 (when the FDA changed its guidelines on DTCA) to more than $4.2B in 2005 (U.S. Government Accountability Office,

Prescription Drugs: Improvements Needed in FDA's Oversight of Direct-to-Consumer Advertising, GAO report Number GAO-07-54, December 14, 2006; Donohue, J. M., Cevasco, M., & Rosenthal, M. B. "A Decade of Direct-to-Consumer Advertising of Prescription Drugs," *N Engl J Med* (2007) 357(7): 673-681). Advertising directly to patients by pharmaceutical companies and medical device companies has markedly changed demand for services. Many of these new medications and services are unnecessary and most are much more expensive than generic medications and other products of proven value. However, many patients are driven by DTCA to demand the more costly alternatives.

Free samples to physicians have been shown to increase the use of expensive new brand name medications rather than less expensive generic equivalents. The US has 81,000 pharmaceutical representatives, one for every 7.9 physicians. Hours spent by physicians on industry supported continuing medical education (CME) programs that often give attendees "honoraria" and other benefits for attendance is greater than that from either professional societies or medical schools. In the US in 2005, an estimated $29.9B to $57B was spent on pharmaceutical marketing (56% for free samples, 25% for drug representatives to talk to physicians, 12.5% for DTCA, 4% on sales people to hospitals, and 2% for journal ads). In Canada in 2004, for comparison, $1.7B was spent on pharmaceutical marketing. In the US about $20B a year could be saved if generics were used instead of brand name equivalent products (Donohue, *et al. N Engl J Med* 2007, cited above).

End-of-life care: End-of-life care is an uncomfortable topic, but for true healthcare reform, it must be addressed. It is difficult to discuss rationally because of strong feelings about the issue. *Politicians and special interest groups demagogue the issue and have made meaningful discussion almost impossible.* In California, the overall annual Medicare expenditures in 2012 were $19.7B for 2,010,957 Medicare beneficiaries. That's $9,779 annually for each beneficiary. However, for the most expensive top 5% of beneficiaries the annual expenditures were $8.5B or $84,293 for each beneficiary (i.e., 43.1% of total expenditures). For the next top 5% of beneficiaries the expenditures were $3.6B or $35,986 per beneficiary (i.e., 18.3% of total expenditures). Thus more than 61% of the total Medicare expenditures ($12.1B and $60,170 per beneficiary) were for just 10% of Medicare beneficiaries. Most of these funds are expended in the last few years of life. The expenditures for the top most expensive 25% of beneficiaries were almost 85% ($16.7B) of the total Medicare expenditures ($33,218 per beneficiary). One of the factors in this expensive care is that providers, patients and families often want to provide all possible care, regardless of cost, discomfort and suffering. This is often the case even when it is not effective in significantly prolonging meaningful life and, therefore, not very humane care.

We cannot decrease the expense of that care unless we make some major decisions about what is appropriate and cost-effective for end-of-life care. Many physicians understand this and their strategic management transitions to more simplified comfort care measures that focus on pain management and decreasing painful and unnecessary interventions. They also focus more on the family and their adjustment to the realities of their loved-one's impending demise. However, many physicians do not want to "give up". They order many studies and interventions and feel compelled to continue heroic measures. This may be because of the physician's training and beliefs, unrealistic patient and family wishes, or fear of medico-legal risk if everything is not done to prolong life. However, end-of-life decisions can be managed appropriately with patient care conferences. These conferences typically consist of a care team (physicians, nurses, social workers, hospice care givers, and other appropriate providers) that meets with the patient and/or family members to clarify the wishes of the patient regarding their end-of-life care. The discussion includes the nature of the patient's illness and expected course, the patient's wishes regarding cardiopulmonary resuscitation (CPR) and being on a ventilator, the drugs to be used for pain and comfort management, and options for hospice support at home with the family.

Legal Risks:

Risks of malpractice litigation: *The risks of malpractice litigation, or more correctly, physicians' fear of malpractice litigation, have markedly increased healthcare expenses by driving the practice of defensive medicine.* Malpractice premiums and numerous related insurance costs have also markedly escalated. In addition, average per capita tort awards (malpractice payments/judgments) increased more than four-fold from 1980 to 2010.

Tort reform and limitation on punitive damages in some states, such as California, have helped to decrease the rate of acceleration of healthcare costs. However, the limitation on these damages in California is being challenged by trial lawyers and other special interests and may be increased again.

It is important to understand that malpractice insurance premiums and judgments themselves are not as big a cost issue as the cost of excessive testing and defensive medicine practiced by many physicians because of their fear of being sued. As an excessively litigious society, our fears are driving up costs because physicians can no longer defend their actions by relying on their expert clinical judgment and following evidence-based medical standards. For example, "atypical" (meaning probably not caused by the heart) chest pain in a 30 to 40 year old man with minimal or no significant risk factors is generally evaluated with multiple expensive tests, even if his risks are considered low. Counseling on risk factors and healthy lifestyles and watchful waiting with follow-up have become inadequate for legal defense against the rare heart attack in such an individual, even if evidence-based guidelines are followed.

Risks of class action suits: Frivolous, unjustified civil action lawsuits that are not based on facts and are driven by attorney advertising are major problems that drive up the cost of drugs, healthcare devices and procedures. The class action suits against Dow Corning and other manufacturers of silicone breast implants are an excellent example. Litigation alleging such harms as cancer and autoimmune disease cost Dow Corning and other silicone breast implant companies billions of dollars throughout the 1990s and put many manufacturers out of business or in danger of bankruptcy. The lawsuits were largely due to aggressive plaintiffs' attorneys and public opinion, not medical evidence (Schleiter, KE, "Silicone Breast Implant Litigation" *Virtual Mentor* American Medical Association Journal of Ethics, May 2010, 12(5): 387-394). After Dow Corning filed for bankruptcy in 1994, the other plaintiffs agreed on a settlement of $3.2 billion (Bernstein, DE. "Review: the breast implant fiasco" *California Law Rev.* 1999, 86(2): 457-510). Subsequent research clearly demonstrated that there was no risk of autoimmune connective tissue diseases associated with silicone breast implants (Gabriel SE, *et al. N Engl J Med.* 1994; 330(24): 1697-1702) or of breast cancer (National Cancer Institute. National Cancer Institute Breast Implant Study, 2010 www.cancer.gov/newscenter/siliconequanda). Silicone breast implants class action lawsuits were enabled by "silicone doctors" who approved women for inclusion in the lawsuits. The American Medical Association issued a Code of Medical Ethics statement on Medical Testimony in 2004 to stress that physicians involved in litigation must testify honestly and without the influence of financial compensation, keeping the interests of patients in mind (www. ama-assn.org/resources/doc/code-medical-ethics/907a.pdf). Medical witnesses must be held to the standard of facts and evidence-based medicine, not their personal "expert opinion". Truly "expert" medical testimony must not be contrary to facts and data (www.quackwatch. com/01QuackeryRelatedTopics/mcslegal.html). Thankfully, the Supreme Court set up Fry-Reed tests to weed out the glib professional witnesses who base their testimony on junk science. This is just the beginning of what needs to be done to reform the abuses of "expert witnesses" and class action suits. There are still "hired guns" that are highly paid for their "opinions" that are not supported by sound evidence. Even qualified experts presenting well-founded scientific perspectives when testifying about matters of public policy may be influenced more by their personal opinions and beliefs about public policy than by the facts on which those policies should be based.

Regulatory compliance risks: Compliance with overly complex laws, rules and regulations related to healthcare practice are a major problem. The Health Insurance Portability and Accountability Act (HIPAA), the False Claims Act (FCA), the Anti-Kickback Statute (AKS), the Physician Self-Referral Law (Stark law), the Exclusion Authorities, and the Civil Monetary Penalties Law (CMPL) are a confusing mess that make it almost impossible for providers to be sure that they are doing everything correctly. This leads to uncertainties and concerns about risks of financial and criminal penalties. It is a major problem when providers are prohibited from collaborating in some instances and encouraged to collaborate in others, and relieved from those regulations in certain circumstances, but not in others. The bureaucratic complexity and the conflicting regulations that are promulgated by these laws are almost impossible to negotiate.

Preventive medicine and failure of personal responsibility for health: As a society, in general, many are not following the healthy lifestyle, wellness and health promotion recommendations that they should—maintaining healthy body weights, exercising regularly, healthy eating habits, smoking cessation, etc. *A large segment of our population has* *lost their sense of responsibility for their own health and the health of their children.* Childhood obesity has more than tripled in the past 30 years. A third of children (age 6-11 years) and adolescents (age 12-19 years) are overweight or obese (http://www.cdc.gov/healthyyouth/obesity/facts. htm). Most people don't worry about their health when they are young and feeling "bullet proof". As individuals and as a society we should begin to take more responsibility for our personal health and the health of our families. No healthcare system will be efficient unless we prevent and manage diseases before they occur or worsen because of unhealthy personal and family lifestyles.

"It is the property of true genius to
disturb all settled ideas"
—Goethe

POTENTIAL HEALTHCARE COST SOLUTIONS

The Robert Wood Johnson Foundation published the shared views of the 18 members of its RWJF Physician Network on Health Care Costs (*Consensus Themes and Recommendations*, Fall 2013). The consensus of those diverse physicians provides good guidelines for consideration in healthcare reform and cost solutions that should be acceptable to most healthcare providers:

1. Payment models must be evidence-based, physician-endorsed, and thoroughly tested.
2. Protecting and creating financial incentives is critical to broad physician buy-in.
3. Meaningful consumer (patient) engagement requires better communication and guidance from physicians, more willingness from consumers, and greater investments in prevention.
4. Improving quality and reducing cost requires a strong health information infrastructure.
5. Major changes in education and practice are needed to help reduce costs.

These are excellent thoughts and reasonable recommendations that most physicians can agree on. We should first review where we are now, and then consider how we can move forward more productively on these issues.

The ACA and comprehensive healthcare reform: The Affordable Care Act (ACA) was supported by the American Medical Association (AMA represents only 20% of American physicians, largely primary care physicians) and the American Academy of Family Practice (AAFP is a primary care physician organization). They each had specific reservations, as did other provider groups and organizations, which drove some concessions and changes in the bill to make it more palatable to some providers, particularly primary care physicians. The AMA supported the individual mandate, health insurance market reform, and the formation of Accountable Care Organizations (ACOs) to better coordinate patient care. The AMA opposed the ACA reduction in incentive payments for quality from 2% to 0.5% and establishing a 2% penalty for not participating in the revised and renamed Physician Quality Reporting System (PQRS); restrictions on physician-owned hospitals; the failure of the ACA to permanently fix the sustainable growth rate (SGR, the "doctors-fix") that sets payment rates for Medicare to physicians; the proposed Independent Payment Advisory Board; the value-based payment modifier based on outcomes, quality, and risk adjustment scores (tools that do not appear to be scientifically valid or accurate) with 5% payment cuts for "outlier physicians"; and Medicare provider enrollment fees. The AAFP supported guaranteed coverage and expansion of access to healthcare, increased payment for primary care services, increased funding for training of primary care physicians, Patient Centered Medical Homes, and health insurance reform, including preventing companies from denying coverage to patients with pre-existing conditions, but had similar reservations as those of the AMA. There were incentives in the ACA for primary care physician support, but the real impact of those incentives has been less clear with the myriad of complex regulations and administrative requirements being generated with ACA implementation.

The *January 1, 2014 ACA deadline for implementation of changes in healthcare insurance has generated major changes in that industry.* In 2011 there were 148 million people covered by employer health insurance and 15 million with individual insurance for a total of 163 million people, more than half of the total population of 308 million (The Henry J. Kaiser Family Foundation "Health Insurance Coverage of the Total Population", 2012. kff.org/stat-category/health-coverage-uninsured/health-insurance-status/). Nationwide, healthcare insurance companies are cancelling millions of policies and the information released in late 2013 is that *the Administration projected in 2010 that half of all private insurance policies would be cancelled because of the ACA.* The number of cancelled policies will far exceed the number of uninsured Americans (49 million) before the ACA. *The ACA mandates are forcing all healthcare insurance policies to be more uniform, comprehensive and expensive.* This markedly limits consumer choice in selection of healthcare insurance. Beneficiaries are no longer allowed options for mainly catastrophic coverage, Health Savings Accounts with options for personal pay and self-insurance, or other health insurance choices based on individual preferences and needs. *Adding many features that patients do not need and do not want is markedly increasing healthcare insurance costs and limiting competition among plans.* Under the ACA the only real differentiator among plans becomes who provides the services (specific hospitals, physician practices and other service providers) that patients must use. It remains to be seen how successful the exchanges will be. We should all be prepared for expected and unexpected problems, even in states where there has been major support for the effort. For example, a Gallup Poll in the summer of 2013 found that more than 40% of uninsured Americans were not even aware that they are required to buy insurance or pay a fine in 2014.

A consistent majority of the country remains concerned about the implementation of the ACA. *The ACA is problematic regarding its costs and its failure to address many of the most important needs for real healthcare reform.* The vast majority of Americans feel that healthcare is already too expensive. It is now clear that the ACA will increase costs much more than was projected. *Despite the expectations of ACA advocates that the ACA would grow more popular after its passage, it has remained consistently unpopular.* A Kaiser Family Foundation Poll in mid-2012 and again in mid-2013 found that 43-44% of respondents rated it negatively. Only 35-37% rated it positively. *Costs of healthcare insurance have skyrocketed with many premiums doubling or even quadrupling since enactment of the ACA.* Healthcare cost sharing by patients has markedly increased. Millions of people are unable to maintain their current healthcare insurance, as they were promised. The limits on the annual cap of out-of-pocket expenses that include deductibles and co-insurance payments will not permit patients and families to elect healthcare insurance plans with lower costs and high deductibles to protect themselves from catastrophic healthcare expenses, while allowing themselves to self-insure and pay directly for routine healthcare. This was a reasonable, cost-effective alternative for generally healthy people and families who wanted more control of their healthcare. These are just some of the major problems, in addition to the Healthcare.gov website problems, in the confusing implementation of the ACA.

A June 2013 poll showed that 66% of people were worried about their healthcare insurance in the future. The July 2013 Twitter announcement of a year delay in the ACA implementation of the major changes in healthcare insurance provided by big businesses until 1 January 2015 was not a good sign. The implementation would have forced many large business employees off their health insurance plans with *the ACA mandate that large employers must provide coverage for their workers or pay penalties. Most Americans are still required to have health insurance or pay a fine after 1 January 2014.*

However, the biggest problem with the ACA is the loss of trust in the Administration (CNN/ORC Poll released November 25, 2013). This loss of trust raises many questions about the future of the ACA in its present form.

It is clear that Americans want healthcare reform, but the ACA is not the reform that was promised or expected. They want reform that will bring down costs and provide better access to high quality healthcare, not increase costs and decrease their access and options for healthcare. *Nevertheless, there are sound provisions in the ACA that should be considered and appropriately implemented.* This will be difficult if there is no transparency, honesty and collaboration from the Administration on the critical issues that should be addressed and resolved. It is possible that *consensus on some of the provisions of the ACA could form the basis for meaningful, bi-partisan compromises* to move the country forward on a much more rational path to true reform. *This will happen only if the American people take the time to better understand some of these complex issues and demand that our Federal and state governments address the real problems with healthcare.*

Accountable Care Organizations (ACOs), Comprehensive Care Organizations (CCOs) and Patient-Centered Medical Homes (PCMHs, Medical Homes): ACOs, CCOs, and Medical Homes are new models of care that are now being facilitated under the Medicare Shared Savings Programs (MSSPs). ACOs are organizations of providers of healthcare (a team of physicians, clinics, hospitals and other healthcare providers) that work together to provide more comprehensive management of patients. There are several models for ACOs. All give providers incentives for improving the coordination, quality and cost-effectiveness of the healthcare they provide. Providers agree to share some financial risk in these programs. The Center for Medicare and Medicaid Services (CMS) has implemented shared savings for successful ACO programs and MSSPs that improve quality and significantly decrease costs for Medicare beneficiaries. ACOs take responsibility for losses in the program as well as savings. MSSPs encourage providers to move from the Medicare fee-for-service program toward an ACO with less financial risk. Advanced Payment ACO models are a further incentive for participants in MSSPs. CCOs and other MSSP models are still fee-for-service based, but there is incentive for shared savings if they demonstrate increased quality and decreased costs.

Medicare ACO Patient-Centered Medical Homes are assigned to Medicare patients based on where the majority of their healthcare expenses are paid—preferably in their community and near their homes. Other healthcare insurance plans, including United Healthcare Group (UHG) and Blue Cross Blue Shield (BCBS), as well as other health plans and organizations have pioneered similar programs. The goal is to decrease costs by providing more comprehensive, coordinated care for all patients, with a particular focus on those with the highest risks and expenses. *The patient-centered whole person approach for wellness and health promotion, combined with improved access to comprehensive, coordinated, high-quality, cost-effective healthcare are the keys to the success of these programs.* CCOs are also programs to improve patient-centered coordination of comprehensive high-quality, cost-effective healthcare, but provide it under the fee-for-service system. Their goals and focuses are similar to those of ACOs.

There is general consensus that we need comprehensive, patient-centered care coordinated by Medical Homes led by primary care providers in their communities. ACOs, CCOs and similar programs may prove to be good models for providing a Medical Home for patients. The goals are to increase the quality of care and patient satisfaction, improve community health, and decrease per-capita costs by improving coordination of care. The strategy is to focus on the most costly patients to try to decrease admissions and re-admissions to hospitals, frequent emergency department visits, and costly complications. *ACOs are designed to give all providers a share in the cost-savings from their implementation, while keeping them accountable for the appropriateness, quality and efficiency of their services.* They base reimbursement on quality and cost-effectiveness of care and give the organization and providers the freedom to build the most cost-effective systems, much like the traditional fee-for-service system. The difference is that ACOs/CCOs provide a strong incentive for the most appropriate, high quality and cost-effective care, rather than for a high volume of visits, tests, procedures and other forms of care that are directly cost-reimbursed. These are good goals, but the implementation must be flexible. There are anti-trust concerns that must be addressed. Allowing the majority of providers in a region to honestly and freely implement these programs, while also preventing abuse of these opportunities, will be a significant challenge. If properly implemented and monitored, the profit motive can drive the efficiency and cost-effectiveness of these programs, but providers and healthcare business interests must be held accountable.

A major problem with ACOs/CCOs is the potential risk to remote areas and rural facilities. Critical access hospitals (CAHs) and their associated rural health clinics (RHCs) have special issues. First, CAHs are more expensive to operate than large urban hospitals and subsidies to CAHs for skilled nursing facilities (SNFs), a major source of revenues that allow them to operate in small rural communities, have been at risk of being reduced. Many CAHs and SNFs in rural communities would not survive significant cuts in Medicare and Medicaid funding. Second, because of economies of scale it is more expensive to care for patients and to perform laboratory and radiology studies and operative procedures in rural hospitals than in urban hospitals or clinics. ACOs and health plans may, therefore, elect to send patients to less expensive urban centers for these procedures, decreasing the care available in rural patients' communities, increasing patients' time away from work and home, and increasing patients' travel costs. Because of inconvenience, many patients in rural communities may avoid or delay care, defeating the goal of ACOs/CCOs. Third, Medicare assigns each patient to a Medical Home based on where the majority of their healthcare is billed. This is a problem for patients receiving most of their care from travelling specialists or specialists who provide services using telemedicine (interactive video visits) and bill from their office in a distant urban area. If the majority of the rural patient's healthcare is billed from an urban area, Medicare will assign the rural patient to a Medical Home in the urban area, not in their rural community. All of these issues put convenient healthcare for patients near their home in rural communities at major risk. One option that should be considered is to use the patient's home address, rather that the billing address of the physician provider, to assign a community Medical Home to rural patients. Fourth, in many rural communities most healthcare services are from midlevel primary care providers. Midlevel providers are nurse practitioners (NPs), physician assistants (PAs), and other ancillary providers. Current Medical Home assignments are based on physician provider billing, not midlevel primary care provider billing. *Rural patients and rural communities should be recognized as different from urban patients and urban areas. Rural patients should have the option for a primary care provider that may or may not be a physician to coordinate care in their community.*

The National Rural ACO (NRACO) is a collaborative effort of nine rural healthcare facilities in California, Indiana and Michigan (physician groups and hospitals—most are served by critical access hospitals (CAHs) with 25 or fewer beds). Its goal is to facilitate development of regional ACOs in underserved areas through coordinated care efforts. The NRACO is approved for the Medicare Shared Savings Program (MSSP) and plans to expand its network throughout the US to support 60 facilities and communities in ACO development in 2014. Its goal is the Medicare Triple Aim of "better care for individuals, better health for the population, and reduced cost per capita" plus financial sustainability for rural facilities by achieving required MSSP quality measures and markedly reducing costs of care for its target populations. It has established a national data bank with Inland Empire HIE (IEHIE), Riverside, California to facilitate data collection, data analysis, reporting and continuous improvement of quality measures, to give timely feedback to providers on quality performance and costs, and support care coordination and evidence-based medicine programs. The NRACO has partnered with Stratis Health, Minneapolis, Minnesota, that has ACO policies, procedures, and programs (including coaching programs) already proven and vetted. These are all efforts that require significant investment, but because of economies of scale of this project, the NRACO expects the costs to be far less than each region would be required to invest to establish such a program on its own.

An important issue with ACOs/CCOs/PCMHs is how patient care will be coordinated. A primary care physician usually coordinates a team of different providers that may include mixtures of primary care physicians, NPs, PAs, other ancillary providers, and specialists. The foundation of these organizations requires implementation of a team-based approach to healthcare, including disease prevention and chronic disease management. I have been providing telecardiology and other telemedicine services to an isolated, small rural health clinic 80 miles north of Ridgecrest in the high desert of California for more than a decade. The collaboration among the NPs and primary care physicians with the specialists providing telemedicine consults for them has been exceptional. The remote primary care providers have learned to handle more complex issues through our interactions. When I get a consult from the NPs I work with, it is almost always appropriate and needs my input. It is also clear from review of their records that they are managing the routine, uncomplicated care of their patients well, ordering the correct tests, and generally making the right decisions about medications. Over the years they have also learned from our interactions and significantly increased their capability to manage significantly more complex and difficult issues, improving the quality of care available in their small, isolated community. The NPs I work with recognize their capabilities and limitations and have always asked for help when they are concerned about a patient. *A team-based ACO, CCO, and Medical Home approach with predominately NPs will work well in isolated rural and frontier communities that have readily available telemedicine support.*

However, major problems with primary care team-based approaches to healthcare must be solved for us to move forward. *First, we do not have an adequate number of primary care physicians to fully implement the coordinated care programs mandated under the ACA.* The US has fewer primary care providers than any other industrialized country—30 per 100,000 patients, compared to 80 for the UK and >150 for France and Germany. To address this shortage, increasing the number of primary care physicians and the use NPs, PAs and other allied health providers (AHPs) have been proposed.

Second, getting primary care physicians and NPs to work harmoniously together is sometimes difficult. Many physicians are concerned about the differences in training between these important ancillary providers, who typically have one or two years post-college training, and physicians, who typically have at least seven years of medical school and residency training after college. Many NPs can provide routine care for straightforward problems, with similar health outcomes, resource utilization and costs as physicians. However, in many cases professional biases, politics and special interest get in the way of effective collaboration. In 2011, the Institute of Medicine (IOM) and the Robert Wood Johnson Foundation (RWJF) initiated an effort to foster better inter-professional collaboration between physicians and nurses. One recommendation was to remove the scope-of-practice barriers that limit NPs and advanced practice registered nurses (APNPs, NPs with additional specialized training) to permit them to practice to the full extent of their education and training. That recommendation generated controversy in many physician organizations. The Council of Medical Specialty Societies (CMSS), that represents multiple physician specialty societies, opposed the IOM/RWJF recommendation. The CMSS did, however, support the expansion of nursing education to help alleviate the critical nursing shortage that is worsening with implementation of the ACA.

Finally, *the lack of adequate healthcare coverage for behavioral health and mental health issues within ACOs/CCOs and Patient-Centered Medical Homes should be specifically addressed.* Mood disorders (mental health problems) rank third in overall healthcare costs, first in work loss costs, and second in total costs (*Community Mental Health Journal* (2004) 40(1): 75-90). Not covering these services is a major public health problem. To solve this issue we should expand health insurance coverage for mental health and increase the use of psychiatric and mental health practitioners, NPs and PAs to provide better access. We should deal with licensing scope-of-practice limitations that are major issues in the ability of these ancillary practitioners to provide services to the full extent of their training, as well as reimbursement for advanced scopes of practice by APNPs trained to manage mental health problems.

We can also reach more people and decrease costs with telemedicine and telehealth applications. Telemedicine is face-to-face interactive video clinical visits and consults with patients at a distant site from a healthcare provider/consultant. Telehealth is the use of telecommunications technology in a broader sense to provide a whole host of healthcare services, including telemedicine, distance learning and education. Better coordination and integration of all healthcare specialty services and mental health services using telemedicine can markedly decrease costs through integrated team-based approaches, with specialists coordinating services through primary care and ancillary healthcare services providers. We should also have the health information capabilities to identify specific patients within service populations that have the most difficult and expensive problems to manage (frequent hospitalizations and re-hospitalizations, frequent emergency department visits, etc.). Focusing on interventions in their communities and homes to meet specific needs can significantly decrease healthcare costs.

One concern is that *hospitals and big healthcare systems (including insurance companies) are primarily leading many of these efforts, because individual physicians and physician provider groups alone cannot afford to implement these expensive systems and recruit all the parties to make them work.* However, more physicians and physician groups are joining or leading ACOs. ACOs must be a collaborative effort among all parties and money should not just go to hospitals, large healthcare systems and insurance companies. If we want to maintain a profit motive system to drive quality and efficiency, and not push our country to a completely centralized healthcare system, we must maintain the proper balance in these efforts—not an easy task.

Although promising, the mid-2013 results of Medicare's test of 32 Pioneer ACOs were mixed. All participants demonstrated improvements on quality measures and 25 of the 32 participants generated savings. Only 13 received shared savings and two were responsible for paying for losses of about $4 million. Nine of the 32 have discontinued their participation in the test program or changed to the Medicare Shared Savings Program as a lower-risk alternative. This announcement occurred in the setting of a rapid increase in Medicare ACOs from 64 in mid-2012 to 195 in mid-2013, and the Medicare announcement in January 2013 that 450 organizations would participate in bundled payment initiatives (ACOs and Medicare Shared Savings Programs).

Another major caution on collaborative efforts like ACOs and CCOs was raised in the article on "Who's To Blame For Our Rising Hospital Costs?" Forbes.com April 3, 2013. Hospital costs in the US in 2010 accounted for $814B, 31.4% of all healthcare expenditures. *A problem with hospital acquisition of independent private physician practices can be an increase in costs of services.* For example, a Nevada patient's bill for an echocardiogram before a hospital purchased the physicians' practice was $373, but increased to $1605 for another echocardiogram after the merger. These are big issues that must be addressed as we move forward with collaboration and coordination in healthcare reform (see Baicker, K, and H Levy "Coordination versus Competition in Health Care Reform" *N Engl J Med* (2013) 369(9): 789-796).

Decrease mass marketing of brand name drugs, medical procedures, and medical devices directly to patients: We should promote generic drugs that are more cost-effective alternatives and in most cases just as effective as brand-name drugs that are more expensive. As discussed earlier, direct-to-consumer advertising (DTCA) of pharmaceuticals is banned in more than 30 other industrialized nations, but in the US, advertising by pharmaceutical companies directly to patients has significantly changed demand for brand-name drugs.

Two related practices are also disturbing and increase the utilization of brand-name drugs and costs. *First, the direct distribution of brand-name drug samples to physicians* to initially give patients free samples and then write prescriptions for those more expensive drugs. As mentioned earlier, of an estimated \$29.9B to \$57B spent in 2005, the pharmaceutical industry investment to promote the use of expensive brand name drugs by physicians was 87% of their marketing budget, almost seven times the DTCA investment.

Second, public policy mandated healthcare quality measures in some cases causes providers to resort to brand name drug utilization not supported by evidence-based medicine in their efforts to meet low-density cholesterol (LDL) and diabetes control standards set by the Physician Quality Reporting System. In patients with coronary artery disease the brand-name drug ezetimibe is often used rather than the generic simvastatin to decrease the LDL cholesterol level below the target of 100 mg per deciliter. Ezetimibe blocks absorption of cholesterol from the intestines rather than inhibiting cholesterol synthesis in the liver, like statins. Simvastatin and other statins have been shown to decrease the risk of heart attacks, but ezetimibe has not. In 2011 US physicians wrote 14.6 million prescriptions (\$2.5B in sales) for ezetimibe products, compared to 98 million (\$391M in sales) for simvastatin. In patients with diabetes, clinicians frequently used brand-name pioglitazone and related drugs (13.8 million prescriptions, \$4.3B in sales), rather than generic metformin (67 million prescriptions, \$1.4M in sales), even though pioglitazone and related drugs have warnings that they can cause or worsen congestive heart failure, have not been shown to improve patient outcomes, and cost more than seven times as much as metformin. More than 500,000 prescriptions were written for rosiglitazone that is banned in Europe and restricted in the US because of safety concerns (*N Engl J Med* 2012; 369: 299-302). Rational, evidence-based healthcare decision-making, including consideration of cost and consequences of different options, should be an integral part of our healthcare system thinking and healthcare reform. Public policy should not enable and drive questionable or poor medical practices to meet bureaucratic "quality" reporting requirements.

A study of different approaches to manage prescription drug benefits compared more than one million Medicare Part D patients using private plans with distinct formularies with more than 500,000 US Department of Veterans Affairs (VA) patients using the VA national formulary. Medicare beneficiaries with diabetes used two to three times more brand-name drugs than a comparable group within the VA, at a substantially higher cost. Medicare spending in this population would have been $1.4 billion less if brand-name drug use matched that of the VA (Gellad, W, *et al.* "Brand-Name Prescription Drug Use Among Veterans Affairs and Medicare Part D Patients With Diabetes: A National Cohort Comparison" *Ann Intern Med.* 2013; 159(2): 105-114.

We should also develop standards-of-practice for application of medical devices and other innovative healthcare technologies and procedures. We should promote applications that are clearly value-added and cost-effective, discouraging those that are not cost-effective.

While limiting direct marketing of drugs and medical devices to patients may not be an acceptable practice in the US, given our emphasis on freedom of expression, we should still strongly consider the alternatives. Freedom of speech and advertising and its influence on freedom of choice by citizens should be balanced by the duty of government to protect us from preventable harms and being misled by inappropriate advertising. We have moved forward with truth-in-advertising laws and drug information with prescriptions, but the government has gone further and has been more intrusive and pro-active in areas that contribute to population health, but are not directly related to healthcare delivery—standards for food, air and water; limits on trans fat; smoke free workplaces; worker safety standards; vaccination mandates, etc. We should consider the risks, consequences and healthcare costs from marketing of drugs and medical procedures directly to the patients, who might not have the information and expertise to objectively evaluate those products. We should also educate patients and families about the risks of overuse of medications and the risks of specific medical procedures, including for example, the overuse of radiology imaging technologies.

We must not stifle innovation and research, but we should do what is right. Drug and device development industries must return a profit on their investments to continue research and development. However, they should not unreasonably drive the demand for expensive brand name drugs and other technologies. We should find a way to avoid distortion of supply and demand in the market and also allow drug and other innovative companies to recover their costs.

Simplify Federal, state and healthcare insurance rules, regulations and reporting requirements, to decrease administrative costs: Simplifying these administrative issues is critical, but difficult. *Bureaucracy never voluntarily simplifies itself and rarely decreases its administrative burden on healthcare and other sectors of our economy and the public.*

When I was Commander of the Wiesbaden USAF Medical Center in Wiesbaden, Germany, in the early 1990s we had unique opportunities that showed me what we could do when we were forced to make rapid changes and could ignore bureaucratic processes that normally tie us down. I took command of the Medical Center in late June 1990 expecting a relatively quiet tour because of the expected announcement that we would downgrade the facility to a contingency (standby) hospital with the drawdown of our troops overseas. However, Saddam Hussein invaded Kuwait on August 2 and the 82nd Airborne was deployed to Saudi Arabia on August 7 to begin the buildup of US Forces in response to the invasion. I was informed on August 10 that war planners estimated a 50:50 chance that Hussein would invade Saudi Arabia by August 20th. If that happened, we were expected to have hundreds of casualties a day aero-medically evacuated to us for care. I called an emergency meeting of our Executive Committee and other key staff to prepare for the potential crisis. We could expect no additional staff or help in this initial response.

To put this into perspective, our facility was a German military hospital constructed in 1939 (taken over by American forces after World War II) that showed its age and had many problems. One whole wing of the hospital had been closed, including most of the Radiology

Department, with asbestos contamination discovered during a recent renovation. We had only three operating suites, eight beds in our Intensive Care Unit (ICU) and three ventilators, and our Emergency Department (ED) was small, among many other problems.

The hospital staff's response to this crisis was a great example of American ingenuity and out-of-the-box thinking that quickly transformed the Medical Center. A bioenvironmental asbestos abatement team opened our closed wing and the Radiology Department was functional again by September 4. We quickly expanded our bed capacity from 185 to 350 with 500 beds in place, plus 200 more in the Amelia Earhart Hotel connected to our compound. The ED was moved to our Aeromedical Evacuation Staging Area to handle large volumes of incoming patients more efficiently. The more than $4.3M in war reserve materials were re-inventoried and additional supplies and equipment were procured, including ventilators. Our ICU capability was rapidly expanded. Two more operating rooms were opened and two OB delivery rooms were upgraded to be operating suites. In addition, two Urology procedure rooms were equipped as minor surgery suites. Nurses were given extensive ICU refresher training. The staff of our large Dental Department was trained for other tasks—dentists who did conscious sedation were put through an intensive course to assist our anesthesiologists and anesthetists, and dental techs were trained to do administrative and other tasks in the Radiology Department. The community also responded with more than 500 Red Cross and other volunteers trained, including local high school coaches and staffs to assist with whirlpool treatments. Our team eventually took care of 3133 Desert Shield and Desert Storm patients, one-third of all patients evacuated from the Gulf. Fortunately, when the Gulf War commenced in January 1991, we had relatively few casualties and we had no difficulty managing them.

With the drawdown of troops from Desert Storm and in Europe in mid-1991, Wiesbaden Medical Center also began its drawdown toward closure. Those processes provided lessons on how bureaucracies can be streamlined and simplified, especially if there is relief from regulations. We implemented Total Quality Management (TQM) and the USAF Surgeon General relieved us from Air Force hospital requirements not mandated by the Joint Commission and other external regulatory agencies. We simplified our administrative and committee structure, decreasing record keeping and reporting requirements. This markedly improved our efficiency without compromising the healthcare we provided (Ferguson E, J T Fogg, *et al.* "TQM in an Air Force Medical Center" *NAHQ Guide to Quality Management*, 1993, Chapter 14: pp. 223-231). We consolidated and cut committees from 43 to 11 and decreased the time and paperwork required. The pages of minutes for those committees were reduced from 92.5 per month in 1990 to five pages per month in 1992. We also implemented a registered nurse quality services analyst (RN QSA) program to coordinate required quality reviews, including concurrent reviews of patients in the hospital which decreased the workload formerly accomplished by committees and providers. Overall these changes significantly decreased the burdens on front-line healthcare providers. The lesson from this example is clear. *Even Federal bureaucracies can be cut and simplified to decrease the administrative burden on healthcare AND high quality healthcare can be provided more efficiently without increasing risks.* Unfortunately we rarely get such opportunities.

Crisis situations and rapidly changing situations sometime allow for more rational and rapid adaptations to (or relief from) overly bureaucratic and counter-productive mandates. How can we try to move forward with prospective, directed approaches to simplifying unrealistic bureaucratic processes and mandates? We should acknowledge that regulators are responsible for setting standards and providing oversight, but we should insist that those processes be cost-effective, essential and not overly prescriptive and restrictive. Regulators should concentrate on information that must be tracked and they should avoid excessive, irrelevant data collection and record keeping, especially when the information adds little value and increases costs. We must have data and information at all levels for effective coordination of healthcare, but those requirements should be simplified and standardized. Providers and healthcare administrators should be given more freedom to structure their individual programs to meet those requirements.

Increase supply of physicians, mid-level providers and nurses: Significantly increase enrollment in US healthcare provider training programs. *Our goal should be to educate and train all the providers we need in our American system.* We should decrease the need for a large influx of international medical graduates to sustain our healthcare system.

Inform patients and families about healthcare choices, with incentives for the most evidence-based, cost-effective choices: *All patients and families should have easy access to clear and understandable evidence-based information on effectiveness of different healthcare options at the point of care, as well as through public education programs.* This must include information on generic drugs versus brand name drugs, imaging technologies, and surgical procedures. Patients should also have the opportunity to actively participate in discussions of cost-effectiveness and individual cost-sharing, as well as risks, benefits and alternatives of each proposed care plan. An excellent evidence-based information source on these issues for both providers and patients is www.effectivehealthcare.ahrq.gov.

The economic value of enabling more choices on healthcare options should be considered. Quality, cost information, and competition can significantly drive down costs. Two surgical procedures have significantly decreased costs over the last decade—lasik surgery and augmentation mammoplasties, surgeries that are not reimbursed by health insurance. Individuals that want those surgeries must decide where to go for those surgeries and pay for them. The free-market system has decreased the costs because individuals have the freedom to find the best value for those procedures. We should consider a more general principle—if patients had more choices and if information on quality and costs were easily accessible, the free market should drive down costs and increase value in our healthcare system.

To further encourage cost-effective behavior we should also lower costs for office visits and urgent care visits with much higher costs and cost-sharing for inappropriate emergency department visits for routine and non-urgent care. We should also require patients to share costs for imaging studies and procedures, even if only a nominal amount, to raise individual and public awareness of costs of care.

Management of end-of-life care: End-of-life care is a societal issue that must be addressed if we are to manage it appropriately and effectively. To do this we should coordinate efforts throughout all segments of communities and across multiple disciplines. We do need a public entity with the authority to discuss these issues and make informed evidence-based medical recommendations about appropriateness of care. Difficult cases can be facilitated by local hospital Bioethics Committees that include community members—already a common practice. Political posturing with cries of "Death panels" and other distortions are not helpful. We need reasoned and fact-based education to encourage rational and humane decision-making that helps patients and family members focus on how to best manage end-of-life care. This should include information and encouragement for patients and families to think through and complete Advanced Directives to clarify their wishes well before end-of-life care becomes an issue.

Balanced mass media education of the public through Federal, state and non-governmental organizations and healthcare insurance companies is critically needed. People need to understand end-of-life healthcare issues. We can do much better if we focus on managing end-of-life care of patients more humanely with family support. We should provide care at home or in non-hospital care facilities with adequate support from nursing, community health workers, and ancillary caregivers. This is more cost-effective care and will decrease the unnecessary burden of excessive end-of-life costs that is often left to families.

The vast majority of Medicare costs are spent on the top 5-10% of patients in the last two years of life. ACOs/CCOs have the potential to improve the quality and cost-effectiveness of end-of-life care and to significantly decrease overall healthcare costs, if their services are implemented appropriately. *The expense of the last two years of life cannot be avoided unless providers, patients, families and society in general are educated about appropriate care for patients in their rapidly declining last years.* This must include simplification of medication and procedure regimens and, when appropriate, a *focus on palliative care and comfort care measures.* Heroic measures and extensive surgical procedures in many of these patients are often not successful in prolonging meaningful life and contribute to additional suffering with minimal, if any, benefit to the patient.

Establishing Medical Homes well before transition to end-of-life care, comfort care, and hospice care has the potential to decrease healthcare costs and improve the quality of care for patients with chronic diseases. This can decrease admissions to hospitals, emergency department visits, procedures, and over-complicated medication regimens. This should be facilitated by advanced health information technologies, including electronic monitoring of vital signs, medications, and other appropriate indicators, and interactive video telemedicine and telehealth visits of patients in their homes by home health agencies and primary care providers.

Physician training in cost-effective, evidence-based medicine: Another major factor related to medico-legal risks is current academic training in evidence-based medicine that focuses on all the differential diagnoses (a comprehensive review of all potential causes) of a problem and all possible tests that are required to exclude those diagnoses. The transition from that academic training mindset (necessary for teaching) to independent practice that requires a focus on the clearly most probable cause or causes must be taught and properly addressed. The cost of testing and alternatives based on the most probable causes and most cost-effective approaches to patient management should become an integral part of training in the decision-making process in academic medical education. This should not be considered an ethical problem. The real ethical problem is bankrupting patients with excessive tests that add little to their outcomes. Medical expenses are the major cause of individual and family bankruptcies (Himmelstein, DU, *et al.* "Medical Bankruptcy in the United States, 2007: Results of a National Study" *Am J Med* (2009) 122 (8): 741-746).

Malpractice/tort reform: Decreasing the costs of healthcare will require extensive medical malpractice/tort reform. As a nation, we should stop *frivolous malpractice lawsuits, particularly large, class-action lawsuits.* Settlements from large class-action lawsuits often go primarily to lawyers, with minimal reimbursement to individual class-action "victims". Tort reform and *limitation of punitive damages* in more states, as they have been limited in California and some other states, *decrease healthcare costs.* Malpractice insurance premiums and judgments themselves are not as important a cost issue as the cost of excessive testing and defensive medicine that could be significantly decreased with malpractice/tort reform.

Another way to address these issues would be *Federal legislation to prohibit or limit the scope of advertising by the legal profession.* If patients have significant malpractice claims, they can always find lawyers. Under the basic theory of recovery, the legal goal is for injured patients to be put back into the same position they were before their injury. Patients should be justly compensated for their injuries, but they (and their lawyers) should not be turned into new millionaires in the process, putting them in a far better position than they were before their injury. We do not need "ambulance chasers" to drive claims by advertisements that encourages patients to consider claims that are questionable and frivolous. The major beneficiaries in these processes are malpractice insurance companies that sell more and more insurance policies at higher and higher premiums (driving up all of our healthcare costs) and trial lawyers, not patients. Prohibiting or limiting the scope of attorney advertising would change these dynamics back to more professional practices and would significantly reduce healthcare costs.

On the other hand, as standard and essential elements of their professional medical practice, physicians have a duty to *clearly explain and document discussions* of medical procedures, their risks, benefits and alternatives to their patients and families. Understanding and accepting those risks should be a shared responsibility of the physician, patient and family. Except in cases of gross negligence or medical error, adverse outcomes from explained and expected risks should not be the total responsibility of the physician. Adverse reactions from medications and other treatments should also be considered shared patient risks. Every patient is complex with a unique genetic makeup, compounding disease processes and many unknown or unclear factors that alter their risks for any medication or procedure. There is *never* 100% certainty that a medication or procedure will be successful in treating a problem without any side effects or complications.

Preventive medicine with education and incentives to make _everyone_ responsible for their own health: We should all take responsibility for educating our children and grandchildren about healthy eating habits, physical activity and treatment of risk factors that can avoid or decrease the risk of diseases. As members of communities and community organizations we should all take more responsibility for developing and maintaining healthy communities and cultures that promote wellness and excellence. This must be a grass roots effort led from the bottom-up by concerned citizens. We have seen time and time again that top-down programs mandated by governmental organizations do not work by themselves. They can provide us with information and healthy choices, but it is up to us as citizens to take the initiative to make our nation healthy—it won't work in any other way. Wake-up America, before it's time for all of us to pay the piper!

As a country, we have had significant success in decreasing coronary artery disease death rates (decreasing death rates per 100,000 by 2/3rd since the 1960s) by recognizing and modifying risk factors and implementing new treatment technologies. These have been achieved by medical research and implemented through a healthcare system that has led the world in innovation. Having been through that transition of coronary heart disease prevention and treatment, I know how difficult it has been to translate such innovations into programs that can be readily understood, adopted and implemented for our large diverse population. When I was growing up in the 1940s and '50s a healthy breakfast was eggs, bacon, pancakes, lots of whole milk to drink, etc. It was not until the 1960s with the publication of the first paper on the Framingham study that it became apparent that there might be problems with such diets. Even in the 1970s, cardiologists disagreed about the blood levels of cholesterol that were considered healthy. I remember Simon Dack, MD, founder and Editor-in-Chief of the *Journal of the American Cardiology* and a founding Fellow of the American College of Cardiology, arguing that there was nothing wrong with having a cholesterol level of 300.

The seminal epiphany for me regarding coronary artery disease risks was in 1984 when I was Chief of Cardiology at Wilford Hall USAF Medical Center in San Antonio and took care of a fighter pilot, Gary Shepard, who was found to have coronary artery disease at age 40. We were nearly the same age and had very similar risk factors and lifestyles. We both had high LDL cholesterols (above 160) and low HDL cholesterols (below 30). Working with Edwin "Eli" Whitney, an internist who subsequently became a cardiologist, Gary pushed for Air Force wide changes in lifestyles and programs to address risks that had caused his problems. Gary and I both improved our cholesterol profiles with niacin and later with statins when they became available in 1985. Gary, Eli, and I worked with others in the Air Force to change cardiac risks and lifestyles, including instituting healthier diets in Air Force dining facilities—a major battle we had was over offering margarine as a substitute for butter (which was much cheaper at that time) and over other healthier food choices. Eli and Gary's efforts later became the foundation for the Air Force Surgeon General's Coronary Artery Risk Evaluation (CARE) Program to promote wellness, disease prevention and healthy lifestyles throughout the Air Force. Those interests lead to the Air Force/Texas Coronary Atherosclerosis Prevention Study (AFCAPS/

TexCAPS), the first primary-prevention trial in a cohort of patients with average LDL cholesterol and below average HDL cholesterol treated with lovastatin, one of the most often cited primary coronary atherosclerosis prevention studies (Gotto, AM, E Whitney, *et al. Circulation* (2000) 101:477-484).

With the National Cholesterol Education Program (NCEP) in 1985, we began making further steps forward with coronary artery disease prevention. The initial guidelines were for treatment with statins to decrease LDL levels to below 160 in all patients and below 130 in high-risk patients. In the last decade NCEP/ATPIII guidelines recommended treatment of LDL levels below 130 in all patients and below 100 in high-risk patients and many cardiologists are now recommending treatment to decrease levels to 60-70 in patients with known coronary artery disease. "Pushing the envelope" on cholesterol management like Gary and I did in 1984 appears to have made a difference for us personally. Gary is now 72 and has had no further coronary artery disease events in the last 30 years. My LDL was 61 (down from >160) and HDL 83 (up from <30) on my latest lipid panel and a recent high-resolution cardiac CT angiography (CCTA) research study documented a coronary artery calcium score of six (very low risk), large coronary arteries with no obstructions and minimal positive remodeling (repair processes associated with plaques). I'm convinced that treating Gary saved my life. My parents both had coronary artery disease in later life and my father had a stroke in his 80s.

The evidence-based medicine guidelines accepted for publication in November 2013 are changing our thoughts again on reducing risks of coronary artery disease (CAD) and heart attacks with wider statin use (Stone, NJ, *et al.* "2013 ACC/AHA Guidelines on the Treatment of Blood Cholesterol to Reduce Atherosclerotic Cardiovascular Risk in Adults" *J Am Coll Cardiol.* 2013;():.doi:10.1016/j.jacc.2013.11.002). Numerous studies have shown the inadequacies of previous guidelines (Akosah, K, *et al.* "Preventing Myocardial Infarction in the Young Adult in the First Place: How Do the National Cholesterol Education Panel III Guidelines Perform?" *J Am Coll Cardiol.* 2003; 41 (9): 1475-1479; Erbel, R, *et al.* "Coronary Risk Stratification, Discrimination, and Reclassification Improvement Based on Quantification of Subclinical Coronary Atherosclerosis" *J Am Coll Cardiol.* 2010; 56(14): 1397-1406; Hadamitzky, M, *et al.* "Prognostic Value of Coronary Computed Tomographic Angiography in Comparison With Calcium Scoring and

Clinical Risk Scores" *Circ Cardiovasc Imaging,* 2011; 4:16-23). The guidelines from the AHA/ACC are a major advance in the application of statins to improve population health by focusing on atherosclerotic cardiovascular disease (ASCVD) to decrease cardiac and stroke risks. This is the biggest change in ASCVD risk management since the 1980s. It will increase the number of people appropriately treated and decrease the number of people inappropriately treated, increasing the cost-effectiveness and quality of care. Although increased statin use will increase the overall costs for preventive treatment, preventing disease versus managing the late complications of disease has the potential to markedly decrease overall healthcare costs.

Numerous groups are working to develop blood test biomarkers for better detection of early ASCVD, including CAD. In the near future these technologies should allow us to more effectively diagnose and treat early CAD in individual patients. Earlier detection and intervention in the ASCVD process in individual patients will delay or prevent development of advanced CAD decades in their future, improving the quality and cost-effectiveness of healthcare and decreasing costs.

I ran long before it was fashionable, starting with the improved track shoes for runners in the 1960s and upgrading as running shoes rapidly evolved and improved. Exercise has always been a part of my life and it was great to see increased interest in running, jogging and other physical activities in the 1970s and 80s. However, we now may be "losing the bubble" on promotion of regular exercise in schools and in our general population. The result has been more obesity, diabetes, hypertension, and other cardiovascular and cancer risks that promise to increase our healthcare costs in the future. Even I am not able to get adequate exercise—age and previous injuries are not always kind to us! If we don't exercise and take care of ourselves, take care of our children, and the general population by promoting and fostering healthy lifestyles, things will only get worse. We should do better educating all segments of our population and driving public policy toward wellness and disease prevention. This is a much more cost-effective solution to our nation's healthcare problems than focusing on treatment of advanced chronic diseases that could have been prevented, or managed better in earlier stages, with preventive medicine and public health programs integrated into comprehensive, coordinated healthcare programs.

On a plane ride, I talked to a healthy, athletic appearing lady who must have been in her early 40's and was reading a cycling magazine. She told me an interesting story about her health. Twenty-six years earlier she had weighed 260 pounds. Her grandparents were all grocers and there was a family culture of overeating. She had lost 130 pounds after reading Ann Fletcher's *Thin for Life* by going on a liquid fasting diet, changing her lifestyle, and exercising regularly. People can change their lifestyle, but it is difficult and it requires both a commitment to change and persistence in maintaining that change. It is especially difficult if your family and socioeconomic culture "pushes" food.

We should recognize that unhealthy lifestyles, lack of exercise, and overeating are both individual and sociocultural issues. We should have educational programs for the general population with a special emphasis on communities with the greatest problems, including underserved communities, to insure that we reach more individuals and families with unhealthy lifestyles. Educating families about healthy diets (adequate consumption of fruits and vegetables and limiting or avoiding high fat, excess carbohydrate, and refined sugar) and programs to encourage overall healthy lifestyles can markedly decrease obesity and disease risk in children, as well as in adults. We should have focused dietary education programs in underserved communities and consider ways to encourage the use of food stamps on healthy food alternatives. This could include issuing at least a significant portion of food stamps (specially labeled food stamps) that could only be used for *healthy and nutritious food purchases*.

In addition, we should adjust all insurance premiums for risks that result from poor health habits. We should increase premiums for smoking, which increases risks for lung diseases and cancer, and obesity, which increases the risks for diabetes, cancer, hypertension and heart disease. The increases in premiums for smokers should be used for smoking cessation and related assistance programs, such as counseling, medications and follow-up visits. The increases in premiums for obesity should be used for education and assistance programs related to healthy food choices, exercise programs, etc. In addition there should be clear incentives to encourage more healthy lifestyles, such as gradual decreases in premiums if patients enroll in these programs and show continued improvement toward decreasing their risks.

"This is a time of enormous challenges
and opportunities for American health care . . . Yet it is
hard for us to find the time to get the information we
need, and when political talking points too often
substitute for accurate information,
we don't know where to go or
whom we can trust to get objective information."
—Molly Cooke, MD, President, American College
of Physicians (e-mail to ACP Colleagues, 9/11/13)

Fix Healthcare System Processes

Our healthcare system should include advanced health information technologies (HIT) that can provide information whenever and wherever it is needed to optimize patient care. Our current system is far too complex, fragmented, inappropriately over-regulated, and simultaneously under-regulated. We should reform the basic processes of healthcare, addressing the problems and issues discussed earlier, before we automate those processes with advanced HIT. Automating an inefficient system will not solve existing problems.

The biggest problem with our current healthcare system is our inability to coordinate high quality, cost-effective healthcare efficiently. This is clearly confounded by the increasing complexity of governmental rules, regulations and administrative requirements, as well as those from healthcare insurance companies. The costs in productivity for mandated quality and satisfaction reporting, among other requirements, are growing. Our focus on quality and cost-effectiveness should not require physicians and their staffs to spend a large portion of their time on excessive administrative and bureaucratic mandates that significantly decrease their time for actually providing healthcare services.

These problems are magnified by the push of the Health Information Technology for Economic and Clinical Health Act (HITECH Act) and the Accountable Care Act (ACA) to implement electronic health record

(EHR) systems and advanced health information technologies that are not adequately interoperable and are plagued with poor usability. Available EHR systems are not optimal for automating established clinical practices (standard provider-patient interactions: clinic visits, hospital visits, etc.). Almost all EHR systems require extensive training and major changes in practice patterns and clinic procedures for their implementation. Although collecting information in EHRs improves patient care, we are trying to integrate and automate processes using EHRs that are not configured to capture all the data required for good documentation.

To systematically address these problems we should first adequately define the issues and engage all stakeholders. Next, we should fix the basic clinical healthcare process problems through simplification, standardization, coordination and integration. Finally we should facilitate those clinical processes with appropriately developed, easily useable and fully interoperable HIT systems.

Wide and unjustifiable variations in quality and costs of healthcare: For example, the costs and quality of diagnostic coronary angiography (coronary artery catheterization) to assess presence or absence of coronary disease and risk of heart attacks vary widely in different hospital referral regions. In a recent study, costs varied from less than $4000 to more than $14,000 with similar quality (Philip, E, *et al., Health Affairs* (2012) 31(9): 2084-2093). Such wide variations are unjustifiable and unacceptable. Evidence-based standardization of healthcare practices to optimize both quality and costs is required.

High and growing administrative healthcare costs: Costs are driven by excessive and counterproductive regulatory requirements imposed by growing Federal, state, county and other bureaucracies. A great example is the new ICD-10 codes, a medical classification list by the World Health Organization (WHO) that is an expansion of ICD-9, currently still in use in the US. The ICD codes stand for diseases, signs and symptoms, abnormal finding, complaints, social circumstances, and external causes of injury or diseases. Used in many other countries, ICD-10 has 14,400 different codes that permit tracking of problems and diagnoses. *The US Clinical Modifications (US ICD-10 CM) increases those codes to 68,000. A Procedure Code System (US ICD-10 PCS) not used by other countries adds another 76,000 codes, for a total of 144,000 codes that healthcare providers* *must deal with.* Even though the deadline for ICD-10 has been pushed back repeatedly, CMS recommends that medical practices prepare for implementation of the new code system. Not only must new software be developed, installed, tested, and proven in practices, but physicians, staff members, and administrators must be trained to use the coding system. They must also develop new practice policies and guidelines, and update paperwork and forms related to the change to ICD-10.

Government Health IT Editor Tom Sullivan interviewed Richard Averill, senior vice president of clinical and economic research at 3M Health Information Systems about the need for this coding ("Q&A: Why the U.S. actually needs those crazy ICD-10 codes" *Government Health IT,* July 23, 2013). The case for more specific diagnostic and procedural data was based on broader population health issues, providing the potential to create actionable information for unique problems like, for example, sports related injuries. ICD-10 was compared to a dictionary. However, posted comments spelled out the problems for providers with this system:

"As a clinician, I have primarily used ICD-9 codes to report diagnoses to third party payors. I anticipate that ICD-10 will be more granular, but ultimately no more relevant to my practice. As noted in this article, a small subset of words in the dictionary do a wonderful job, make it possible to have a conversation. The really interesting thing is that the words in that unabridged dictionary also make it possible to describe in a clear and meaningful way the patients I encounter in my practice.

Yes, I find it hard to be enthusiastic about learning and using codes to replace clear and concise English prose, especially when the main purpose of the coding seems to be to allow computers to deny payment if diagnoses and services fail to align in a master table."

"The plethora of codes will confuse. Confusion will produce bad data. I so hope that an improved ICD-11 comes within a year and is introduced to slim the code set.

There is an "infographic" with amusing 10 codes. I actually checked each of the ten and found them accurate. But these were in an area where someone(s) bureaucratically made each code symmetrical. Some of the codes are simply moronic.

This will eventually doom the attempts to make ICD-10 accepted by the physicians and other providers who will be the users. Coding clerks will not be able to take records and produce proper codes without recourse to the provider for several minutes per patient about many patients."

US ICD-10 CM and PCS are going to be difficult, if not impossible, to sell to providers. Such unreasonable bureaucratic requirements are just compounding the difficulties for providers to coordinate with multiple payers with different rules, regulations, fee schedules and documentation requirements. The only answer is *simplification and standardization of administrative processes*. This will only occur if we cut the bureaucracies, forcing regulators and bureaucrats to concentrate only on what is critical and most important for optimizing the cost-effectiveness and quality of healthcare. This will mean reducing many regulatory requirements and the size of the bureaucracies that are perpetuating them. It will also mean adding some regulatory requirements, particularly related to more efficient and effective coordination of care. The simplification and standardization of administrative healthcare processes, coupled with adequate HIT applications, will improve the ability to track quality and cost-effectiveness of care. Abuses, waste and inappropriate processes in our healthcare system can also be identified more easily if processes are simplified.

Legal risks:

Malpractice risk: Providers should have significant protection for their professional judgment if they are following evidence-based guidelines to provide high quality and cost-effective care. Major costs of malpractice litigation are legal fees and the size of malpractice awards. Some states have already made significant tort reforms to limit unreasonable punitive damages. All providers, to some extent, practice defensive medicine to decrease their risk of malpractice claims.

Coronary artery disease (CAD) is a great example. It is the single largest killer of Americans, with one acute coronary event every 26 seconds and one death every minute. The most common presentation for CAD is an acute myocardial infarction (heart attack) or sudden death in someone who previously had no indication of disease. These events occur with rupture of a vulnerable soft plaque that would not have been detected by routine stress testing, EKGs or nuclear studies. Even invasive cardiac catheterization (coronary angiography) can miss vulnerable plaques. They often cause less than 30 to 50% narrowing of a coronary artery before they rupture, completely occlude the vessel and cause a heart attack. Currently we do not have adequate blood tests to detect early coronary disease. Unfortunately, 50% of the men and 65% of the women who present with heart attacks are previously apparently healthy with no symptoms until the event. The current guidelines by the American College of Cardiology and American Heart Association are to implement general preventive measures (smoking cessation, control of hypertension, treatment of high cholesterol, management of diabetes, etc.), wait for symptoms (generally late disease with a >60-70% blockage in a coronary artery) or wait for an acute event (heart attack) that is often fatal. These are the evidence-based guidelines that we now follow.

Our ability to reliably diagnose early atherosclerotic cardiovascular disease is limited. Preventive measures initially instituted in the 1970s through the 1980s and more recent measures have made a difference. More aggressive treatment of risk factors has markedly decreased the number of people in the US dying from acute coronary events. However, unsuspected acute coronary events in patients that have previously been evaluated for chest pain are still a major problem. Physicians are put at medico-legal risk even if patients were managed according to evidence-based guideline.

So how do physicians in Emergency Departments (EDs) respond to the hidden problem of asymptomatic CAD? Anyone who presents to the ED with any symptoms that might be cardiac in origin is subjected to a full workup to try to determine, *first* if they are having a heart attack, then if they are not having a heart attack what their risks are for a heart attack. This frequently includes multiple EKGs, radiology and laboratory studies, hospitalization, nuclear stress tests, and even transport for diagnostic cardiac catheterizations. In the US in 2007 this strategy for atherosclerotic cardiovascular disease (the vast majority being CAD) resulted in 6.2 million surgeries and procedures, and direct and indirect costs of $286 billion. Much of this expense is driven by a focus on late disease and procedures. A significant contributor to this cost is defensive medicine. To assure ED physicians that they do not send anyone home that has not been thoroughly evaluated, even patients who obviously have non-cardiac and musculoskeletal chest pain, have multiple tests because of the small risk that they will later return with an acute coronary syndrome (heart attack).

One answer is to improve our capability to evaluate chest pain and manage different stages and risks of CAD in EDs with improved technologies. A study of 4691 patients presenting to EDs with a diagnosis of chest pain that was not clearly an acute coronary syndrome or non-cardiac chest pain, demonstrated that CCTAs decreased hospital admission rates from 40% to 14% (Poon, M, *et al.*, *J Am Coll Cardiol* (2013) 62:543-52). Standard evaluation without CCTA increased the length of stay in the ED by 55% and was associated with a 7-fold greater likelihood of invasive coronary angiography without revascularization (diagnostic cardiac catheterizations). The improvement in quality and cost-effectiveness of care with this approach is obvious. In addition, since this study was done in large metropolitan hospitals, the impact of quality and cost-effectiveness of care in isolated rural hospitals should be even more profound.

Legal compliance risk: Excessive rules and regulations, the time and expense of complying with all of them, concern about the risk of substantial fines or other legal actions for missing one of a myriad of requirements can substantially decrease the cost-effectiveness and efficiency of healthcare. A clear illustration of the risks involved in legal compliance is the US Department of Health & Human Services Office of the Inspector General publication *A Roadmap for New Physicians: Avoiding Medicare and Medicaid Fraud and Abuse* (http://oig.hhs.gov/fraud/PhyscianEducation/). After praising physicians in general, the following is the conclusion of the Introduction:

"The presence of some dishonest health care providers who exploit the health care system for illegal personal gain has created the need for laws that combat fraud and abuse and ensure appropriate quality medical care. This brochure assists physicians in understanding how to comply with these Federal laws by identifying "red flags" that could lead to potential liability in law enforcement and administrative actions. The information is organized around three types of relationships that physicians frequently encounter in their careers: I Relationships with payers, II Relationships with fellow physicians and other providers, and III Relationships with vendors. The key issues addressed in this brochure are relevant to all physicians, regardless of specialty or practice setting."

The publication then goes on to say in the Fraud and Abuse Laws overview:

"The five most important Federal fraud and abuse laws that apply to physicians are the False Claims Act (FCA), the Anti-Kickback Statute (AKS), the Physician Self-Referral Law (Stark law), the Exclusion Authorities, and the Civil Monetary Penalties Law (CMPL). Government agencies, including the Department of Justice, the Department of Health & Human Services Office of Inspector General (OIG), and the Centers for Medicare & Medicaid Services (CMS), are charged with enforcing these laws. As you begin your career, it is crucial to understand these laws not only because following them is the right thing to do, but also because violating them could result in criminal penalties, civil fines, exclusion from the Federal health care programs, or loss of your medical license from your State medical board."

In that section it makes clear that under the False Claims Act (italics and underlining added)

"**It is illegal to submit claims for payment to Medicare or Medicaid that you know *or should know* are false or fraudulent.** Filing false claims may result in fines of up to three times the programs' loss plus $11,000 per claim filed. Under the civil FCA, each instance of an item or a service billed to Medicare or Medicaid counts as a claim, so fines can add up quickly. The fact that a claim results from a kickback or is made in violation of the Stark law also may render it false or fraudulent, creating liability under the civil FCA as well as the AKS or Stark law.

"*Under the civil FCA, no specific intent to defraud is required.* The civil FCA defines "knowing" to include not only actual knowledge but also instances in which the person acted in deliberate ignorance or reckless disregard of the truth or falsity of the information. Further, the civil FCA contains a whistleblower provision that allows a private individual to file a lawsuit on behalf of the United States and entitles that whistleblower to a percentage of any recoveries. Whistleblowers could be current or ex-business partners, hospital or office staff, patients, or competitors.

"*There also is a criminal FCA* (18 U.S.C. § 287). *Criminal penalties for submitting false claims include imprisonment and criminal fines.* Physicians have gone to prison for submitting false healthcare claims. OIG also may impose administrative civil monetary penalties for false or fraudulent claims, as discussed below."

The Anti-Kickback Statute section states (italics and underline added)

"The AKS is a criminal law that prohibits the knowing and willful payment of "remuneration" to induce or reward patient referrals or the generation of business involving any item or service payable by the Federal health care programs (*e.g.*, drugs, supplies, or health care services for Medicare or Medicaid patients). Remuneration includes anything of value and can take many forms besides cash, such as free rent, expensive hotel stays and meals, and excessive compensation for medical directorships or consultancies. **In some industries, it is acceptable to reward those who refer business to you. However, in the Federal health care programs, paying for referrals is a crime** . . . . *Under the CMPL, physicians who pay or accept kickbacks also face penalties of up to $50,000 per kickback plus three times the amount of the remuneration.*

"Safe harbors protect certain payment and business practices that could otherwise implicate the AKS from criminal and civil prosecution. To be protected by a safe harbor, an arrangement must fit squarely in the safe harbor and satisfy all of its requirements. Some safe harbors address personal services and rental agreements, investments in ambulatory surgical centers, and payments to *bona fide* employees."

The Physician Self-Referral Law section states (italics and underlining added)

"*The Physician Self-Referral Law, commonly referred to as the Stark law, prohibits physicians from referring patients to receive "designated health services" payable by Medicare or Medicaid from entities with which the physician or an immediate family member has a financial relationship, unless an exception applies.* Financial relationships include both ownership/investment interests and compensation arrangements. For example, if you invest in an imaging center, the Stark law requires the resulting financial relationship to fit within an exception or you may not refer patients to the facility and the entity may not bill for the referred imaging services.

"Designated health services are: clinical laboratory services; physical therapy, occupational therapy, and outpatient speech-language pathology services; radiology and certain other imaging services; radiation therapy services and supplies; durable medical equipment and supplies; parenteral and enteral nutrients, equipment, and supplies; prosthetics, orthotics, and prosthetic devices and supplies; inpatient and outpatient services.

"*The Stark law is a strict liability statute, which means proof of specific intent to violate the law is not required.* The Stark law prohibits the submission, or causing the submission, of claims in violation of the law's restrictions on referrals. Penalties for physicians who violate the Stark law include fines as well as exclusion from participation in the Federal health care programs."

The above passages are just an overview of the first sections of this pamphlet. They were included in some detail to give readers a feel for the complex bureaucratic and legal constraints physicians, hospitals and healthcare systems must follow to adjust their practices to assure that they either comply with or get specific exemptions from Safe Harbor clauses.

A recent case highlighting this problem is a judgment against Tuomey Healthcare System, a 240-bed hospital in Sumter, South Carolina, for $277 million (Carlson, J, *Modern Healthcare,* October 1, 2013). The issue involved more than 21,000 Medicare claims worth a total of $39.3M. The court imposed $39.3M in Stark penalties and $237.5M in False Claims Fines for an institution with total annual revenues of $202M. A local physician "whistleblower" had filed a Federal lawsuit alleging that

19 contracts with specialty physicians in the area violated the Federal ban on compensating doctors based on volume and value of patient-business they referred.

Additional risks that healthcare providers face are audits, sanctions and fines for HIPPA personal health information (PHI) violations, EHR meaningful use incentive audits, and IRS revenue code violations. There are also challenges for payments and reasonable compensation that require documentation of how provider (primarily physician) compensation was determined, including clear job description, services and duties; third party support for compensation; exceptions and safe harbor issues; fair market value; and compensation cap.

The CMS Recovery Audit Contractor (RAC) Program has a mission of identifying and recovering improper Medicare payments. Private contractors are hired to find any faults they can in claims paid in the past five years (increased from three years) to recover payments. *Claims can be reviewed based on current standards, not standards at the time of claims.* Auditors can recover >$1B/year and are getting more aggressive in their audits. Audits can include charge master, coding, processes (revenue cycle and patient flow), specific type of service or code (evaluation and management codes, therapy codes), internal policies and processes (patient transfers and bed assignment), code pairs and related modifiers, hospital inpatient admission order certification (record must be completed, signed, dated, and documented prior to discharge; must have 2-midnight stay *after the admission order is documented*; authorization must be signed by physician responsible for the case or a physician knowledgeable with the case). Hospitals and providers are also being held responsible for mistakes made by independent companies that are contracted to submit claims, even if due diligence has been done and adequate compliance procedures confirmed.

The lack of CMS oversight of Medicare Zone Program Integrity Contractors (ZPICs) who perform RAC audits and the lack of knowledge and expertise of ZPIC staffs has been a major problem. Many providers have closed their practices or lay off employees because of aggressive actions taken by ZPICs based on poorly conducted investigations. In most of these cases, no fraudulent activity was identified and cases were never referred for legal action. However, Medicare reimbursement was withheld and the huge amounts of money, time and energy required for providers to defend these actions have ruined many legitimate providers and their practices (van Halen Group, LLC "Bipartisan effort to combat waste, fraud and abuse in the Medicare and Medicaid programs", White Paper Submission to the Senate Finance Committee, 2012; Fletcher, D. "ZPICs—The Most Dangerous Weapon in Medicare's Arsenal" http://www.nrrts.org/business-articles/ zpics-the-most-dangerous-weapon-in-medicares-arsenal).

Overregulation and excessive, complex and confusing documentation requirements and overzealous enforcement activities greatly increase healthcare costs. *The risk of being unable to comply with every detail of these bureaucratic requirements is undermining our American healthcare system and driving many providers to leave the practice of medicine.*

Anti-trust risk: Accountable Care Organizations (ACOs) proposed by the ACA are designed to coordinate care within a region by developing business and collaborative arrangements among hospitals, providers, healthcare systems and other partners in a region. The goals are to improve quality of care, cost-effectiveness of care and overall population health in the region served. Setting up these organizations is problematic without anti-trust exemption and some relief from or clarification and adjustment of compliance regulations cited above, as they apply to ACO implementation.

Most patients and the general public are not aware of these legal and regulatory constraints on hospitals, physicians and healthcare systems. As somewhat of an aside, physicians have been forced to make changes over the last 40 years—the court mandated change in professional ethics to permit open advertising of services; more concentration on the business of medicine but with constraints that prohibit or severely limit many common business practices; increased regulatory, legal and administrative record keeping and reporting requirements, etc. Yet now physicians and hospitals are being pushed for more collaboration and coordination of care to be built on sharing of revenues for cost savings among providers and hospitals. Providers can't deal adequately with conflicting mandates that both inhibit and promote collaboration in business practices that are essential to provide higher quality and more cost-effective care.

As you read this, if you are confused about some of these issues, join the crowd. Physicians and administrators in clinics and hospitals live with these constraints and spend millions of dollars in attorney fees and on other measures to assure that they and the businesses they work with are in compliance. There are reasons for oversight and constraints, but we should consider the costs of compliance requirements and the inefficiencies that they induce in our healthcare system. It is difficult to live with uncertainties about the risks of any action that could result in major fines or imprisonment because of misinterpretation or inadvertent mistakes.

Evaluating and implementing new technologies and systems of care: Providers, payers and regulators must work together to evaluate and appropriately guide the use of expensive new drugs, equipment and procedures, as well as new models for providing care. This must include cost-effectiveness, as well as efficacy, and must be soundly based on evidence-based medicine.

Implementing ACOs may play an important role in more effectively guiding our healthcare processes. Lessons from the Pioneer ACOs were instructive. Alicia Caramenico ("4 Lessons from Pioneer ACOs," FierceHealthcare.com, September 24, 2013) reported that one of the Pioneer ACOs that elected to change from the ACO to the Medicare Shared Savings Program model cited four specific lessons: *First, Focus on Data*: Predictive analytics allows identification of patients that need special attention, who can be identified through data aggregation and connectivity. *Second, Engage Patients*: Work with community organizations (churches, nonprofits and poverty programs) to make entry into ACOs easier for patients. *Third, Rethink Emergency Care*: Consider implementation of geriatric emergency departments for patients ≥65 years of age—those with a high percentage of complex issues. *Fourth, Expand Workforce*: Hire more nurse practitioners to identify patients at risk for admission and re-admission; care managers to coordinate care; mental health guidance counselors or facilitators to coordinate with psychiatrists; nurses to improve health system navigation and chronic disease management; health and wellness coaches; data managers. Only with such coordinated approaches can we reach the triple aims of improving population health, improving the experience of care and decreasing per-capita costs. I would add two more points. *Fifth, Implement Clear Evidence-based Guidelines: Standards of care and care plans should be clearly defined for providers to use and for patients to more easily understand and follow.* Require development of appropriate guidelines and educational programs for both providers and patients. Getting providers to agree on these guidelines and adhere to them may be difficult, until we have adequate data and health information analytics to evaluate individual provider actions and compare their actions with those of other providers with regard to quality and cost-effectiveness. *Sixth, Simplify Physician Tasks*: Give physicians and other providers the tools to document their work faster, more intuitively, and consistent with the way they are trained to practice medicine, not systems that slow them down and require extensive modifications in their normal practice. Coding, billing, quality of care assessments, and other administrative data should flow automatically from their basic visit and procedure records without any major interventions on their part.

To implement effective ACOs and other healthcare technologies, *further development and implementation of comprehensive evidence-based guidelines is critical. We, as a nation, should have HIT systems to measure evidence-based guideline implementation and effectiveness at the individual provider and individual facility level. That information will help drive truly meaningful and rational healthcare reform.*

Stakeholders: Providers of healthcare services and goods, governments, regulators, payers and administrators are all obvious stakeholders in healthcare. By far the largest stakeholder group is the population served. Beneficiaries/patients should be involved in all of the above processes to give them "skin in the game" and let them help guide this reform: *First, beneficiaries should be made aware of the wide and unjustifiable variations in healthcare quality and costs in their region.* This will force the needed improvements in the quality and costs of care. *Second, patients should be informed about the exceptionally high and growing administrative and overhead costs imposed by excessive regulatory requirements* that are driving up the cost of their care. They are already aware of the dysfunctional leadership from our Federal and many of our state governments that is driving up their personal healthcare costs, their taxes, and the national and many state debts. *Third, patients should be informed about the evidence-based medicine options for their personalized care plans to play a more critical role in the decision-making process.* They should be informed about the costs, risks and benefits of each option. *Fourth, patients should be appropriately educated about the application and the misuses of expensive new technologies.* Patients should have unbiased information about those technologies, instead of getting most of their information from mass media advertisements, drug and procedure vendors, and others who have a major stake in pushing the technologies. *Fifth, all patients should also be given a stake in the game by being required to pay a cost-share for most of their healthcare services and choices.* The ACA does this by requiring approved plans to have cost-sharing for healthcare services—40% for Bronze plans, 30% for Silver, 20% for Gold and 10% for Platinum. Another option to consider is giving patients more choices with plans that include reference pricing which is another type of cost-share by patients (Reinhardt, U. E., "The Sleeper in Health Care Payment Reform" Economix, *The New York Times*, August 2, 2013). Reference pricing is a very powerful way of controlling costs by local and regional providers and hospitals. Patients are required to pay the difference between a reference price and what providers and hospitals charge. With open and transparent information for patients on quality and costs, where there are provider options and large variations in quality and prices, providers and hospitals would be forced to compete by increasing quality and decreasing costs.

The basic tenet is that all patients and families must have an increasing role in healthcare decision-making. They must be better informed about their options to allow them to make personal selections about their care. This will also give them a major stake in efforts to reform the healthcare system. To accomplish this effectively, patients and families should have access to information on standard costs and ranges of costs for medical procedures and drug treatments to allow them to make more informed decisions. Patients are beginning to get unbiased, clear information on both quality and costs from multiple sources (see "Your safer-surgery survival guide" ConsumerReports.org September 2013, as an example).

In addition to improvements in quality and cost-effectiveness of healthcare for ill patients, *a major national and community focus must be on health promotion and wellness education.* We will never reach our goals for the health of our country until our national leadership and all segments of our population focus on major education programs for all citizens and residents, particularly underserved communities. This must include non-partisan programs supported by political leaders, healthcare and community organizations, educational institutions, news and public service media and all other venues to stimulate significant changes toward more healthy lifestyles in every community.

Simplification: Our uniquely American healthcare system can be adequately reformed through simplification and standardization followed by improved coordination and integration of services. Significant simplification of laws, rules, and regulations is required. One step in simplification should be more standardization of fee schedules for healthcare insurance companies and possibly even coordinated by a single payer system. Once we address the current and growing complexities of our healthcare system processes and correct them, we can markedly decrease the administrative costs of healthcare delivery—the major problem we face. This will require systems that are simpler and more intuitive for providers and patients.

Standardization: We should appropriately standardize administration and delivery of healthcare services to support high quality, cost-effective, evidence-based medical care. In the larger healthcare context, this should include education programs to promote public health, preventive medicine, and wellness promotion for all individuals and communities. This should also include management based on population databases that can identify individuals with high risks who need particular focuses of attention. Reducing wide variations in quality and costs of healthcare services can only be accomplished with data that can be collected, evaluated and acted upon nationally, regionally and locally.

Coordination: We need much better coordination of care among providers with implementation of PCMHs within patients' communities and coordinated by regional CCOs, ACOs or similarly structured programs. This would be a major advance toward providing comprehensive care more efficiently and at lesser cost.

The issue of coordination of care versus competition to decrease costs in healthcare reform should be addressed. ACOs and bundled payment programs focus on better coordination of healthcare, but integration of systems of providers may encourage anticompetitive practices. Quality reporting, price transparency, and pay for performance can improve coordination and competition by focusing on quality, value and cost-effectiveness of care. We can strike the right balance by working with regulatory agencies and courts that enforce antitrust laws to implement policies that foster the optimal quality of healthcare while allowing competition to keep the cost of care as low as possible (Baicker, K, and H

Levy, "Coordination versus Competition in Health Care Reform" *N Engl J Med* (2013) 369(9): 789-91).

Integration: Eventually we must move to better integrate services. Initially this is a process problem as we learn through coordination of services within and through PCMHs, CCOs, ACOs and other organizations. Developing agreements that coordinate all these functions among diverse patients, providers, clinics, hospitals, payers, etc. is a daunting task. To become truly integrated we must have comprehensive electronic health record (EHR) systems coupled by advanced HIT that allow seamless health information exchange. To be successful in these programs we must have real-time accesses to EHRs, laboratory data, radiology images, interactive video telehealth applications for assessing patients, interaction with consultants, patient portals, easy access to wellness and health promotion guidelines, and other healthcare information. Data analytics to evaluate the performance of individual providers and individual hospitals, clinics, and healthcare systems are also essential to maintain our focus on healthcare quality and cost-effectiveness. This will enable assistance to providers and systems that need improvement and rewards to those that provide high quality, cost-effective care.

In summary, our goal is to provide all segments of our population access to affordable, high quality, cost-effective, patient-centered healthcare options. We should increase our focus on wellness and health promotion programs to decrease long-term risks of disease though more healthy life-styles. We must coordinate these efforts with integrated broadband HIT systems. We should maintain financial incentives for building competitive, high quality, cost-effective healthcare systems at all levels (national, state, regional, local, individual provider and individual patient). Bureaucratic and legal barriers should be reformed to permit open and secure access to standardized health information data. Functional, integrated, health information data exchange systems are key to the success of our reform efforts. *Everyone must have a stake in the game.*

Implement health information technologies: HealthIT.gov provides excellent reviews of health information technologies (HIT). It includes explanations of the benefits of HIT, definition of terms and other essential information for providers and professionals, patients and families.

Government HIT implementation programs should be acknowledged for their positive benefits. The Health Information Technology for Economic and Clinical Health (HITECH) Act, part of the American Recovery and Reinvestment Act (ARRA) of 2009, rapidly pushed electronic health record (EHR) and other supporting HIT adoption by physicians and hospitals. The HITECH Act provided $19 billion to support meaningful use adoption of EHRs, $2 billion to establish the Office of the National Coordinator (ONC) and support the implementation of the HIT infrastructure necessary for health information exchange (HIE), direct funding for HIT in Federally Qualified Healthcare Centers (FQHCs), Indian Health Service facilities, and other related support funding. These investments, including the Broadband Technologies Opportunities Program (BTOP), and other investments to support HIT, total more than $30 billion and are one of the largest infrastructure investments in our country's history. They have rapidly moved many HIT capabilities forward to support healthcare. While there is much concern expressed regarding the expense and effectiveness of the ARRA, the HITECH Act and other programs have greatly accelerated EHR adoption and have helped us move towards development and implementation of meaningful HIE. To further clarify terms, HIE is the transmission of healthcare information using telecommunications systems, such as the Internet or other IT networks. EHRs (also called EMRs) are electronic health/medical records that store the information previously entered into paper charts that providers use for healthcare records. "Meaningful use" of HIE is the ready electronic access of health information from EHRs to support healthcare decision-making.

The history of HIE efforts over the last few decades should be understood in the context of ACA implementation. Consumer driven community health management information system (CHMIS) grants were not successful in implementing sustainable centralized community databases in the early 1990s. They were not affordable and the technology was inadequate. Community health information networks (CHINs) later in the 1990s also failed because they were commercially driven decentralized networks that were competitive, not community stakeholder driven and had unsustainable fees. Regional health information organizations (RHIOs) and HIEs in the 2000s had difficulty establishing sustainable business models. However, in passing and implementing the ACA, the Federal government envisioned a future of low cost, high quality healthcare enabled by the rapid adoption of advanced HIT (Vest, JR, LD Gamm "Health information exchange: persistent challenges and new strategies" *J Am Med Inform Assoc* 2010; 17:288-294). The strategy focused on personal health records and the individual consumer, employment of healthcare institutional incentives and regulations (HITECH act and EHR adoption), the HIE as a public good to benefit everyone, and reliance on technology innovations. This strategy now appears to be significantly flawed because standards for interoperability (above HL7) and the business value proposition are inadequate to allow us to move forward.

Najeeb Al-Shorbaji of the World Health Organization (WHO), gives an interesting perspective applicable to our current struggles on the issues facing implementation of universal healthcare strategies in different countries around the world:

> "(There are) . . . common elements, methodologies and best practices that can help countries avoid mistakes, for example, investing large amounts of money without a proper plan, roadmap or a strategy—this leads to fragmentation wasting resources, disconnection with people and 'solutions looking for problems' . . . Absence of timely and quality health data simply means hasty decision-making, non-evidence-based planning, low and delayed care delivery, opinion driven management . . ." (Zack McCartney, "Health IT takes hold around the world" *Healthcare IT News* October 24, 2013 www. healthcareitnews.com).

Rich Swafford, who manages the national data repository for the National Rural ACO, echoes all the precautions noted above and knows the difficulty of this undertaking:

> "I think it is important to note that the development and use of HIE in the US is still very new. The market is immature and the development of business strategies towards the adoption of HIE are still very much in development. Further, the foundation of the ACO model from a data perspective is really based on HIE deployment and as such has some growing to do as well."

In the summer of 2009, there were major concerns about the Federal government throwing so much money at HIT implementation before adequate infrastructure and standards were in place to move forward. Automating systems without clearly defined standards and automating inefficient healthcare processes were major risks. However, despite some major uncertainties and difficulties, many positive changes occurred. *First, organizations that had not and would not work together in the past rapidly realized that this process was much bigger than any one organization could lead.* In California, we formed the California Health and Human Services (CHHS) eHealth Coordinating Committee to get us all working together. New members from leadership positions in various organizations were added to different Boards to facilitate the collaborative process. *Second, the push for interoperability forced EHR and other HIT vendors to move toward common standards that were required for certification of their products*—although EHR systems and other HIT systems are still far from true interoperability. *Third, many resources were developed to support the education of healthcare providers, HIT specialists and other personnel necessary to begin the integration and maintenance of EHR, HIT and HIE systems.*

Significant HIE challenges include not just implementation of infrastructure and sustainability of business models, but specific issues with technology capability. Another major issue is still how we manage both the security of patient information and its ready availability to healthcare providers. HIPPA issues must be addressed and significantly modified toward the correct balance. We should consider different levels of security for compartmentalizing different categories of data based on risks—for example, Level I (highest level) for patient identification information linking name, social security number, date of birth, etc.; Level II for billing and financial information; Level III for specific individual clinical information; and Level IV for general population demographic information.

Other issues are how we develop the technologies to adequately use and analyze the data (new data analytics techniques). Analysis of structured data, such as clinical laboratory results that can be searched and trended for individual patients, as well as for groups of patients and populations in data banks, is one issue. A bigger issue is unstructured data, such as histories, physicals, reports, letters, etc. that are text. Searching that data is more complicated, but is necessary for finding information on specific patients and for converting that information to structured data that can be trended for individual patients, groups of patients and for population management.

Ultimately, the unifying solution after implementing truly interoperable and user-friendly HIT systems will be the building and efficient use of the interstate electronic information highway system for seamless HIE. In the 1950s, President Dwight Eisenhower led development of the interstate highway system that completely transformed our nation's transportation system. That system connected all parts of our country and was a boon for our economic development. We now need an interstate highway system for HIT funded by public-private partnerships. Making such a system work is not only difficult, but it is expensive and it will require that all of us work together. We still have a long way to go regarding usability of EHRs and interoperability of systems, a major source of physician and other healthcare provider frustrations.

The vision: The Office of the National Coordinator (ONC) for Health Information Technology, *Principles and Strategy for Accelerating Health Information Exchange (HIE)* was published in August 2013, and sets a vision for moving forward with these tasks. The report makes it clear that access to individual patient-level health information is essential for healthcare reform and for improving the quality, efficiency and safety of our healthcare system. It outlines a two-step process for achieving meaningful interoperability of health information systems: First developing the capability to *exchange information* among systems, and then developing the capability to *use that information* in a meaningful way. This will require implementing common standards and overcoming numerous usability problems that are currently major issues with HIE.

Solutions and challenges with implementation: Since enactment of the HITECH Act of 2009, adoption of EHRs in the US has markedly increased. Key findings in a RWJF report (DesRoches CM, Painter MW, and Jha AK (Editors), *Health Information Technology in the United States: Better Information Systems for Better Care,* Robert Wood Johnson Foundation, 2013) include:

- In 2012, 40% of office-based physicians adopted at least a basic EHR.

- Half of physicians found that generating lists of patients by lab results or need for overdue care, to track referrals or reports on quality of care was very difficult, somewhat difficult, or impossible.
- 44% of hospitals had at least a basic EHR, up more than 17% since 2011 and nearly tripled since 2010.
- Only 5% of hospitals could meet all 16 of the core objectives for stage 2 meaningful use; however 63% met 11 to 15 of those objectives.
- 30% of hospitals and 10% of ambulatory practices sent and received data through HIEs.
- Test results and patient care summaries were the most common electronic data exchanged (82% and 79%, respectively), while public health reports were the least common (30%).
- HIE efforts continue to struggle financially with 74% of HIEs identifying development of sustainable business models a moderate or substantial barrier.
- Improvements were needed for tailored, EHR-enabled patient education at the point of care and through patient portals (Internet websites). Particular challenges included readily accessible information that was linked to specific patient needs and appropriate for patients with low literacy and limited English proficiency.

These findings show substantial progress, but leave no doubt that we still have a long way to go for meaningful use of EHRs and HIE. The ONC report also makes it clear that there are even greater problems in HIE implementation in post-acute and institutional long-term and post-acute care, behavioral care, and laboratory facilities that were not eligible for Medicare and Medicaid EHR incentive programs. Only 6% of long-term care facilities, 4% of rehabilitation hospitals, and 2% of psychiatric hospitals have even a basic EHR system (Wolf L, J Harvell, A Jha, "Hospitals Ineligible for Federal Meaningful-Use Incentives Have Dismally Low Rates of Adoption of Electronic Health Records" *Health Affairs* (March 2012) 31:3505-513). In addition, about 40% of Medicare beneficiaries are discharged from acute care hospitals to skilled nursing facilities or rehabilitation hospitals that have little capacity to support

HIE functions (Bogasky, S, *Post-Acute Care Episodes Expanded Analytic File*, April 2011).

The California Healthcare Information Partnership and Services Organization (CalHIPSO, the largest Regional Extension Center for EHR adoption) completed a market research survey of EHR/HIE issues and needs in the summer of 2013 for development of a Health Applications Platform (HAP). The HAP was a joint effort with the California Telehealth Network to integrate services, improve interoperability of EHRs with other HIT/HIE systems and facilitate more meaningful use of healthcare information. A focus group of 32 participants and 168 online survey respondents that included physicians, clinical staff, supervisors, executives, and technology directors gave their feedback on EHR implementation, adoption, utilization and other issues. Satisfied users cited portability, efficient workflows and team collaboration, ability to capture data, and chart legibility, but there were frustrations with EHRs regarding loss of productivity, slowness, decreased number of patient visits and systems not being user-friendly with too many clicks. It was interesting that in a state that has made a major effort to implement the ACA, only 51% of users surveyed were currently sharing electronic patient information, including laboratory data and radiology images with other physicians or hospitals and 42% were still planning to or would like to share that information in the future, while 7% did not even want to share electronic patient information in the future.

A discussion in the CalHIPSO Physicians Advisory Council was revealing. Members noted that some providers and groups had decided that there was no good business case for true meaningful use of HIE (penalties cost less than implementation costs), implementation of HIT over inefficient processes is problematic, there are major problems with usability of EHR systems, and there continue to be major interoperability and integration issues with diverse EHR vendors. One member cited a study on "Rapid Usability Assessment of Commercial EHRs" that was presented at the American Medical Informatics Association. Expert EHR users evaluated meaningful use tasks with five of the most commonly used EHR systems and documented that the time to perform the tasks was high. They detected 1266 usability problems in the EHRs. Clinical summaries, computerized physician order entry (CPOE) and e-Prescribing had the highest number of usability problems. The conclusion of the study was that "Poor usability is a critical challenge that will limit the adoption and safe use of EHRs" (Walji, MF, *et al.* AMIA Abstracts 2012: 1665).

The July 2013 Black Book "State of the EHR Replacement Market" report on the research survey of nearly 2900 practices found that 413 of 520 qualified EHRs scored less than midpoint scores in usability of basic functions (see PRWeb ebooks). The survey concluded that there are expectations for new comprehensive EHR technologies that are easier to use. Replacement market EHR buyers are now looking for more intuitive, friendlier systems that do not decrease and may actually increase productivity.

Usability problems have been recognized for years, but have not been adequately addressed. Cedars-Sinai Medical Center in Los Angeles, California spent $34M on implementing an EHR system that was launched in 2002 and abandoned within three months (Connolly, C. *Washington Post*, March 2005). In 2009, the year the HITECH Act was enacted to drive EHR adoption rapidly, the Healthcare Information and Management Systems Society (HIMSS) concluded that the key reasons for slow adoption were, not only costs and lost productivity, but the lack of efficiency and usability of EHRs (HIMSS EHR Usability Task Force, "Defining and Testing EMR (EHR) Usability" HIMSS, June 2009). In 2011, the National Institute of Standards and Technology (NIST) of the Department of Commerce released a study on EHR usability and documented that EHR vendors attempts to develop interfaces only made usability issues proliferate (NIST, "Technical Evaluation, Testing and Validation of the Usability of Electronic Health Records" September 2011). In 2012, a KLAS study reported that half of provider practices that already had EHRs were planning to replace them because of lack of functionality and support (KLAS Research "Ambulatory EMR 2012: Market Splitting Under Adoption Pressure" June 2012).

The SK&A "Physician Office Usage of Electronic Health Records Software" report May 2013, listed 20 EHR vendors with the major market shares (10.6% to 0.8%) and 422 other EHR vendors with a total of 26.3% of the market share. Only three vendors had >10% market shares (Allscripts, eClinicalworks, Epic) and the next ten had 6.1% to 1.9% market shares (NextGen, Practice Fusion, GE, McKesson, Cerner, AmazingCharts, AthenaHealth, Greenway, MedPlus, e-MDs).

Building the interstate highway system for HIT connectivity will not solve the major problems with EHRs and HIE. We must have a complete transformation of how we are currently using EHR systems. Future EHR/HIE systems must be intuitive and easy to use and have the capability to be interoperable with all other EHRs/HIEs, patient management and business systems. These new systems will undoubtedly include iPads, tablets, mobile apps, remote patient monitoring, enhanced connectivity, true interoperability, revenue cycle management, evidence-based medicine decision support, comprehensive population management, patient portals, cloud storage, custom workflows and many other features to simplify EHR use and enhance speed, quality and cost-effective, value-based care. New systems designed around the patient interaction processes that physicians and other providers routinely use to provide care must be intuitive and simple to use in order to streamline processes. They must also support managers, payers, patients and all stakeholders. The ultimate goal is to have a product that allows providers to evaluate patients more efficiently in the same amount of time or in less time than they could see them before the transition from paper and pen to computer AND to provide their services with higher quality, lower costs and better patient satisfaction and outcomes.

One of the good things and one of the bad things about EHRs are exactly the same, the capability to review 10-20 times the information available at each visit. Positive aspects are readability of records, guidance with coding decisions and expedited scheduling and front office procedures, including billing. Providing Health Summaries for patients (problems lists, allergies, medications and past histories) and for other providers and e-Prescribing are also major benefits that clearly improve care.

A new generation of EHRs that are built with markedly improved interoperability and enhanced usability based on how physicians actually perform a patient visit is arriving on the market. Some of these new applications will prove to be disruptive, transformational technologies that if left to open market forces will completely change the current fragmented EHR market.

"If you want to go fast, go alone.
If you want to go far, go together."
—African Proverb

ROLES AND SOLUTIONS FOR HEALTHCARE REFORM

Critical role of the will of the people: We, as individuals, must maintain our freedom of choice for our healthcare. We should have options for healthcare that are adequate and support our needs. *We the People must demand accountability of our Federal and state government leadership for all of their actions that are contrary to our interests and our will.* This is particularly important regarding interests and will to improve the efficiency and cost-effectiveness of our healthcare system. To do this we should be well-informed and involved in simplification of our healthcare system. We cannot just be bystanders. *Healthcare providers, payers for healthcare, Federal, state, county and local governments, non-government organizations and media organizations have a duty to share unbiased information to educate the public on these issues.*

Role of Federal and state governments: Federal and state governments, besides simplifying the complexity of our healthcare system by decreasing its administrative burden, can markedly improve our healthcare system by guiding and supporting the appropriate implementation of comprehensive advanced HIT. The ultimate goal should be the true meaningful use of EHRs, HIE and other HIT to allow the secure exchange of clinically meaningful information among providers nationwide to support high quality, cost-effective healthcare.

Role of healthcare insurance companies and other big businesses: There are major uncertainties for healthcare insurance companies and related businesses in the current economy and regulatory climate. However, many healthcare insurance companies and other healthcare related businesses have made major progress toward improving quality of care and increasing cost-effectiveness of healthcare through competitive healthcare reform efforts.

The Blue Cross and Blue Shield Association is a national federation of the 37 Blue Cross and Blue Shield (BCBS) plans in all 50 states, the District of Columbia and all US territories. They have programs with provider partners in market or in development in 49 states, the District of Columbia and Puerto Rico that include Pay-for-Performance Plans, PCMH, Episode-Based Payment, and ACOs. The BCBS PCMH in Michigan saved an estimated $155M and lowered adult ED visit rates by 9.3% and use of high tech imaging by 8.3% in 2011; Horizon PCMH lowered Medicare hospital readmissions by 25%, hospital inpatient admissions by 21% and decreased costs by 10%; BCBS Advocate ACO of Illinois reduced readmissions for chronic conditions by 26%, reduced hospital admissions 10.6% and decrease ED visits by 5.4% in the first six months of 2011 compared with 2010 (Share, D.A., and M.H. Mason, *Health Affairs* (2012) 31(9): 1993-2001; Choudhri, A, "Payor-Provider Collaborations: Care Delivery and HIT, eHealth Initiative Webinar, September 12, 2013).

United Healthcare Group (UHG), in its recent publications *A Playbook for States: Seeking to Modernize their Health Care Systems* and *FAIRWELL TO FEE-FOR-SERVICE? A "Real World" Strategy For Health Care Payment Reform* (Working Paper 8, December 2012), outlines some rational and appropriate suggestions that are worth reviewing. The *Playbook* outlines strategies for providing healthcare options, modernizing public programs to ensure access to affordable high-quality care, adopting patient-centered innovations to promote better health and drive quality outcomes, and leveraging innovation and technology to build a modern and effective 21st century healthcare system. The Working Paper discusses what is wrong with fee-for-service payment and how measuring the quality and efficiency of healthcare and giving feedback can facilitate continuous improvement and decrease costs. UHG's Premium Designation program has been evaluating physician performance on quality and efficiency in 21 different fields of medicine since 2005 and provides information to patients, providers, employers and other plan sponsors to promote better and more cost-effective (value-based) healthcare.

This program covered one-third of practicing physicians (250,000 physicians in 41 states) with analysis of more than 75 conditions/diseases using more than 300 specific measures of quality care. In this program 43% of physicians were designated as providing quality and efficiency of care and another 14% for quality only. Designated physicians that were recognized for the quality and cost-effectiveness of their care had improved outcomes compared with their peers and national standards. Medicare's "Physician Compete" program and web site that provides similar evaluations is of limited utility and does not provide comparisons of performance of specific physicians. Medicare's "Hospital Compare" program and web site has similar problems and demonstrates little or no improvements in the treatment of heart attacks, heart failure or pneumonia. *Programs that are built by and for providers are much more successful than government driven programs that are implemented without adequate input from providers.*

Other healthcare plans and healthcare systems have pioneered similar quality programs to those described above. All of these programs focus on features that should meet the following goals for quality, efficiency and transparency. First, they should be clearly defined, evidence-based, and acceptable to the providers. Second, they should have a minimal administrative burden for their evaluation and measurement. Third, they should be uniform and focus on high-value measures. Fourth, they should be allowed to evolve over time with experience and evidence-based data. In addition, those programs and insurance plans should provide more choices and options for individual consumer/patient services and cost structures than are currently allowable under the ACA. The ACA is undermining many better options.

Essential Role of Providers: Physicians and other healthcare providers are the keys to any viable healthcare reforms. They must be given a widespread and prominent role in the reform process. They are the experts at actually providing care and services directly to patients—not Federal and state government bureaucracies, health insurance companies and third party payers, and big healthcare businesses. However, in the current ACA healthcare reform process, providers are generally being demonized and are not being given a significant voice.

Physicians and other front-line providers must be permitted to get back to *the profession of medicine.* They know how to provide high quality, cost-effective healthcare that satisfies patients and keeps our population healthy. They should be relieved from excessive, expensive and overwhelming governmental regulatory requirements and from fears of inadvertent non-compliance and sanctions that could destroy their practices.

Our governmental institutions, in particular, should have more collegial, cooperative and supportive interactions with front-line providers. If we are to implement PCMHs with physicians leading coordinated care teams to provide higher quality, more cost-effective care to patients, physicians should have a prominent role in the development of the laws, rules, regulations and policies that govern healthcare entities. Truly effective and meaningful healthcare reform will not be achieved without greater collaboration with physicians and other providers.

Provider payment reform: Provider payment reform depends on the options we choose: Pay-for-performance and care management initiatives with adjusted fee-for-service payments to reward quality and efficiency, such as PCMHs; Bundled or episode-based payments with a fixed sum to cover all costs of services for an episode of care; Shared-savings and shared-risk approaches, like ACOs and other MSSPs; Capitation payments with fixed fees to providers for services to all patients under their care

Pay-for-performance and care management initiatives: United Healthcare Group (UHG) implemented the Practice Rewards program in 2006 and expanded it to 27 states. The program rewards physicians who meet defined quality, efficiency and administrative criteria with higher fee-for-service payments. This program and similar programs in the public and private sectors found limited to modest improvements in quality care. Based on their experience, UHG developed a larger-scale program, Performance-Based Contracting (PBC), for contracting with physicians and hospitals. Most contracts by 2014 will include an annual increase in payments based on performance measures.

The PCMH is another model where all patients receive comprehensive, coordinated, and patient-centered care. Preliminary results of PCMH pilots have shown gross savings on medical costs of 4.0-4.5% per year and net savings (with additional payments for care coordination and bonuses) of about 2% with notable improvements in care quality measures

Bundled and episode-based payments: Bundled payments give providers incentives for controlling costs because if costs differ from the payment, they keep the savings or pay the excess costs. This approach needs incorporation of adequate quality metrics and incentives to address population health and avoid episodes.

Optum's Centers of Excellence program has more than 20 years experience using this model in treating patients with solid organ and stem cell transplants for congenital heart disease and with other rare conditions. These conditions are treated in highly specialized centers and Optum developed a comprehensive approach to drive quality and efficiency. Optum's Centers of Excellence were able to:

- Improve transplant one-year mortality rates 3% for liver transplants and 5% for heart transplants
- Decrease average length of stay 25% for transplants
- Reduce the incidence of transplants 16% with application of evidence-based appropriateness criteria
- Save an average of 49% per case compared with billing charges for transplants

(Ortner, N J, *2005 US Organ and Tissue Transplant Cost Estimates and Discussion*; and Hauboldt, RH, *2007 US Organ and Tissue Transplant Cost Estimates and Discussion* (Brookfield, WI: Millman, Inc.).

UHG's pilot program for episode-based chemotherapy payments is working with five medical oncology groups on new payment models, with a focus on best practices and better health outcomes. The rationale for this program was two-fold: First, wide variations exist in chemotherapy regimens for common cancers both across and within oncology practices. Second, large revenues for oncology practices come from "mark-ups" on chemotherapy drugs, not on professional services. Studies have shown opportunities to decrease costs and improve outcomes (Neubauer, M A, *et al.* "Cost Effectiveness of Evidence-Based Treatment Guidelines for the Treatment of Non-Small-Cell Cancer in the Community Setting", *J Oncology Practice* (2010) 6(1): 12-18; Newcomer, L N, "Changing Physician Incentives for Cancer Care to Reward Better Patient Outcomes

Instead of Use of More Costly Drugs" *Health Affairs* (2010) 31(4): 780-85).

The Medicare program has led the use of bundled payments since introducing them for inpatient admissions in 1983. Under the ACA, the Center for Medicare and Medicaid Services (CMS) has proposed several bundled payment models that are still being considered and refined.

Shared-savings and shared-risk approaches: ACOs are shared-savings and shared-risks organizations of groups of providers that agree to take responsibility for quality and cost performance for a defined population. If they can improve quality of care and reduce total costs, they can benefit from the savings. Recent experience with ACOs has been mixed and most have shown increases in quality, but marginal or no decrease in costs, as previously discussed.

ACOs and bundled payment programs focus on better coordination of healthcare, but integration of systems of providers may encourage anticompetitive practices. Quality reporting, price transparency, and pay-for-performance, on the other hand, can improve coordination and competition by focusing on quality, value and cost-effectiveness of care. HIT can enable both coordination of care and competition through quality reporting and price transparency, but only if they enable meaningful use of interoperable EHR systems. This is a major problem that has not been adequately solved. Again, the goal is to reach universal capabilities for HIE to allow access to healthcare information when needed for healthcare decision-making on individual patients. (See Baicker, K, and H Levy, "Coordination versus Competition in Health Care Reform" *N Engl J Med* (2013) 369(9): 789-91 for an excellent review of these issues).

Capitation payments to providers: Capitation arrangements encourage physicians to work together to optimize care and reduce variations in practice patterns by taking full financial risk and accountability for a defined population—a population-based payment. This approach has significant drawbacks as 60% of physicians feel that capitation payments shift too much risk to providers and only 20% think that capitation payments encourage appropriate medical care.

"Even if you're on the right track,
you'll get run over if you just sit there."
—Will Rogers

Conclusion and Recommendations

The American people clearly want rational healthcare reform. We also want our leaders to focus on our interests and our needs, not their own special interests and their bureaucracies. We should hold them accountable in every election for their actions. We should not accept the attitudes of some Federal and state leaders and bureaucrats that they work for those systems and not for us. We should make a concerted effort to focus our elected and appointed leaders on healthcare issues that most of the American people can agree on, including:

- Individual freedom of choice in health insurance coverage,
- More universal healthcare insurance coverage,
- Insurance for pre-existing conditions,
- Implementation of advanced HIT systems,
- More efficient systems of care to improve coordination of our personal healthcare, including health promotion and wellness programs for disease prevention, with documentation of quality and cost-effectiveness of care,
- Transparency of information regarding costs and options for services and procedures to allow patients to make more informed decisions.
- Convenient and timely access to healthcare providers that provide quality healthcare, where we can choose a provider as easily as we can choose a good restaurant using an "app" on a smart phone.

We should address the increases in costs of healthcare and the decreased options for health insurance with the implementation of the

ACA. The increases in costs are driven by mandates for inclusion of "essential" benefits that many do not want or need. Our freedom of choice in those different options should be maintained.

We should not concede that we should move from fee-for-service to a fully capitated system for healthcare. Many of the options for more coordinated care that promote improvements in healthcare quality and cost-effectiveness through competition and financial incentives have been developed by different healthcare service businesses (private health plans, health insurance companies, hospital systems, etc.). They provide potential paths forward in reforming our healthcare system in a more reasonable way than are many of the legislative and administrative mandates of the ACA.

With more than 40% of low-income adults being under the age of 65, we cannot ignore the needs for reform. The bi-partisan Medicaid expansion and reform plan of Michigan is an excellent framework for more rational, cost-effective healthcare reform linked to free market incentives and innovations (Ayanian, JZ "Michigan's Approach to Medicaid Expansion and Reform" *N Engl J Med* 2013, 36; 19: 1773-1775). It is based on five core principles: *First*, the state must have sufficient cost-savings from the plan to offset its contributions for Medicaid expansion when Federal funding for Medicaid decreases from 100% to 95% in 2017 and to 90% in 2021. *Second*, financial incentives for new Medicaid enrollees are designed to limit inappropriate use of healthcare services and to encourage adoption and maintenance of healthy behaviors and lifestyles. This includes cost sharing for new enrollees with annual incomes between 100% and 133% of the Federal poverty level. The cost share is as much as 5%, increasing to 7% after 48 months on the new program, but the cost sharing can be reduced to as low as 2% if enrollees demonstrate that they are following healthy behaviors. *Third*, the state will enroll new eligible adults in private health plans, rather than fee-for-service Medicaid. Reimbursement of private health plans will be based on achieving cost and quality targets and health plan sharing of cost-savings based on the clinical value of services provided, much like the ACO model. *Fourth*, new enrollees must have access to primary care and preventive services. They will also be given the opportunity to complete Advanced Directives to encourage early discussions and decisions regarding end-of-life care. *Fifth*, the capability of the state to monitor the costs and quality of care will be enhanced. This includes a new Health

Care Cost and Quality Advisory Committee to promote transparency of data that should help evaluate and improve evidence-based decision making for all parties in their healthcare system.

The bottom line on healthcare reform is to keep the good attributes of our uniquely American healthcare system intact and correct the inefficient aspects of our system by:

1. Addressing and correcting the wide and unjustifiable variations in healthcare quality and costs;
2. Decreasing the exceptionally high and growing administrative and overhead costs of healthcare;
3. Enabling providers to practice more efficiently and more cost-effectively by
   a. Decreasing the time required for tasks not directly related to healthcare services,
   b. Simplifying and streamlining the usability of EHRs and other HIT,
   c. Simplifying and automating reporting requirements, and
   d. Decreasing the risks (malpractice risk and legal compliance risk) for providers that use their medical judgments and follow evidence-based medicine guidelines for patient care;
4. Developing teams of providers, payers and regulators to more effectively evaluate and guide the use and application of expensive new drugs, equipment and procedures;
5. Involving more providers and patients in the decision-making processes of healthcare reform.

The rational implementation of advanced HIT systems will allow coordination and integration of our healthcare systems. This has the potential to provide healthcare information whenever and wherever we need it to make healthcare decisions on individual patients. It should also provide information to allow patients, providers, payers, regulators, and other partners in our healthcare system to focus on high-quality and cost-effective healthcare. For this to be successful, we should first fix or replace EHRs that fail usability and interoperability criteria. We should migrate to EHR systems that are interoperable, built on open architecture, and support the clinical processes that physicians learn in their medical training. These new systems should be intuitive, user friendly, and cost-effective to enhance productivity, rather than decreasing it, as current systems do.

For successful healthcare system reform, we should also build and maintain incentives for quality, evidence-based medical practice, efficiency, cost-effectiveness, and team-based coordination of care. We should focus on avoidance of hospitalization of many complex patients with management problems by coordinating care in their homes and community, as well as health promotion and disease prevention to improve the health of the general population. Providers and all healthcare system stakeholders must be given the opportunity to profit from building and operating systems that provide high quality healthcare more efficiently and cost-effectively. The proper incentives can greatly increase the value that patients receive from their healthcare experiences.

The ultimate goal of rational healthcare reform is a financially sustainable healthcare system that provides high quality, cost-effective care to all citizens through optimal healthcare for each individual in our nation.

Abbeviations

ACA—Affordable Care Act of 2010
ACO—Accountable Care Organization
ARRA—American Recovery and Reinvestment Act of 2009
AMA—American Medical Association
ASCVD—Atherosclerotic cardiovascular disease
ATP III—Adult Treatment Panel guidelines for treating cholesterol in healthy people
BCBS—Blue Cross Blue Shield
CAD—Coronary artery disease
CAH—Critical Access Hospital, limited to 25 acute care beds
CCTA—Coronary computer tomography angiography
CCO—Coordinated Care Organization
CHHS—California Health and Human Services
CMS—Center for Medicare and Medicaid Services
CPOE—Computer Physician Order Entry
CT—Computer Tomography
DHHS—Department of Health and Human Services
DPH—Department of Public Health
DTCA—Direct to consumer advertising
ED—Emergency Department
EHR—Electronic health record
EMR—Electronic medical record (same as EHR)
FDA—Federal Drug Administration
GAO—US Government Accountability Office
HDL—High-Density Lipoprotein cholesterol associated with low cardiovascular disease risk
HIE—Health Information Exchange
HIPAA—Health Insurance Portability and Accountability Act
HIT—Health Information Technology
HITECH Act—Health Information Technology for Economic and Clinical Health Act, enacted as part of the American Recovery and Reinvestment Act of 2009
HMO—Health Maintenance Organization

ICD-10—International Statistical Classification of Diseases and Related Health Problems (ICD) 10ᵗʰ revision of a medical classification list of the WHO

LDL—Low-Density Lipoprotein cholesterol associated with increased risk of heart disease

MSSP—Medicare Shared Savings Program

MRI—Magnetic resonance imaging

NASA—National Aeronautics and Space Administration

NP—Nurse Practitioner

OECD—Organization for Economic Cooperation and Development

ONC—Office of the National Coordinator for Health Information Technology

OSHPD—Office for Statewide Health Planning and Development in California

PA—Physicians Assistant

PBC—Performance-Based Contracting

PCMH—Patient Centered Medical Home

PCNP—Primary Care Nurse Practitioner

PCP—Primary Care Provider

PHI—Personal health information

UHG—United Healthcare Group

USAF—United States Air Force

US ICD-10 CM—US Clinical Modifications of ICD-10

US ICD-10 PCS—US Procedure Code Modification of ICD-10

WHO—World Health Organization

ACKNOWLEDGEMENTS

I owe this book to many mentors who taught me and gave me opportunities. To my father, the most understanding, wise and caring man I have ever met. I still miss him and his counsel. To my mother, a strong disciplinarian, and my grandfather Reuben "Papa" Wilson, my early childhood father figure, a rancher in rural south Texas. They raised me while my father was in World War II in Europe and later at Clark Air Force Base in the Philippines. They gave me a strong-willed, independent "Wilson" heritage. To my high school track coach Clark Massey, who taught me to work hard and to aspire to be better than I had the talent to be. Leadership and the high, competitive standards of teachers like him are essential for the successful development of the youth of our country. To Dr. Pat McKee, who taught me the rigors and discipline of research and scientific writing. To Dr. Jay Sanford, founding Dean and then President of the Uniformed Services University of the Health Sciences, Bethesda, Maryland, who selected me to be the Acting Chair of Biochemistry and to participate in the establishment of the University, giving me diverse opportunities to learn and develop.

To my brother Bill and his wife Kitty, both rural primary care physicians. To the numerous healthcare professional organizations I've worked with to improve rural healthcare. To James Suver, MHA, CEO, and the staff and providers at Ridgecrest Regional Hospital, the critical access hospital where I practice in the isolated, remote high desert of California. They have taught me great lessons about American healthcare and its enormous challenges, particularly how to provide healthcare in remote, underserved areas.

In writing this book I also must acknowledge numerous reviewers and contributors. First is my wife, Dr. Sun Paik. She is the consummate editor, proofreader, fact checker and literature researcher. I'm indebted to many who have reviewed and commented on the book from a variety of different perspectives: Ruth Cooper, JD, Emeritus Board Member, Ridgecrest Regional Hospital; Katy Jo Lynch, MD, PhD, MPH, rural practitioner in North Carolina; Eric Brown, President/CEO, California Telehealth Network; Rich Swafford, PhD, Executive Director, Inland Empire Health Information Exchange; Les Gawlik, JD, Baltimore, Maryland; John Faltys, Med-RT; Sajid Ahmed, CIO, Martin Luther King, Jr. Hospital—and others, too many to name, who have contributed to the process of writing and thinking through the difficult issues discussed in this book.

About the Author

Dr. Earl W. Ferguson, MD, PhD, Col USAF MC (Retired) is a healthcare executive, cardiologist, and preventive medicine specialist with a major interest in cardiovascular imaging, telemedicine, telehealth, telecommunications and computer applications to healthcare. He is a Fellow of the American College of Cardiology, the American College of Physicians and the American College of Preventive Medicine. He is CEO of Sun BioMedical Technologies that he and his wife, Sun Hye Paik, PhD, DPharm, founded in 2002 for research on inflammatory diseases, including early, undetected atherosclerotic cardiovascular disease. He is coordinating development of Cardiovascular Imaging and Coronary Artery Risk Evaluation (CARE) Programs at Ridgecrest Regional Hospital and Coordinated Cardiovascular Care in the high desert region of Southern California.

He provides cardiology consults to Ridgecrest Regional Hospital and its Rural Health Clinic. He also provides telemedicine consults to remote areas of the high desert of California and remotely monitors patients with pacemakers and automated implantable cardiac defibrillators. He is Medical Director, National Rural Accountable Care Organization, and Executive Director of the Southern Sierra Telehealth Network established in 2001. He has served on numerous boards, including the California State Rural Healthcare Association, California Broadband Cooperative (Digital 395 Project), California Telehealth Network, California Health Information Partnership & Services Organization, Ridgecrest Regional Hospital, and National Space Biomedical Research Institute External Advisory Council. He was on the Editorial Board, Telemedicine and eHealth Journal for almost two decades.

Dr. Ferguson was a member of the Federal Senior Executive Service as the Director of Aerospace Medicine and Occupational Health for NASA before moving to Ridgecrest in 1996 to develop advanced rural health information technology applications. He has been in public service his entire career, spending most of his Federal service career in academic and leadership positions, including commanding and supervising large healthcare systems, hospitals and medical centers.